"At last! A measured approach to 0-3's viewing of moving image media that does not impose screen-use rules, but reveals a closely observed world, opening our eyes to the many ways in which babies and infants interpret and enjoy moving images."

Lydia Plowman, *Professor Emerita, University of Edinburgh, UK*

"Bazalgette offers fascinating insights into children's moving-image experiences: a refreshing and important alternative to 'screen time' rules. Based on meticulous research and years working with teachers and parents, this book will appeal to a wide general readership."

David Buckingham, *Honorary Professor, UCL Institute of Education; Emeritus Professor, Loughborough University, UK*

Beyond Screen Time Guilt

Beyond Screen Time Guilt: The Role of TV and Video in Early Child Development by Cary Bazalgette offers a fresh and insightful perspective on babies' and toddlers' relationship with moving image media. Forget the guilt-inducing screen time rules and dire warnings about developmental harm – this book reveals what's really happening when your little one is captivated by their favourite show.

Drawing on meticulous observational research and 35 years of media education expertise, Cary Bazalgette uncovers the remarkable ways in which children under three actively engage with film and television. Bazalgette critiques the flawed research behind screen time rules, exposing the limitations of surveys and experimental studies in this context. She provides vivid examples of typical behaviours, such as spontaneous laughter, frightened responses, and apparent "addiction," while analysing the learning challenges that young children eagerly embrace. The book also emphasises the value of shared viewing experiences and offers detailed insights into how specific TV episodes foster learning.

With its clear style, good humour, and evidence-based reassurance, *Beyond Screen Time Guilt* is an essential read for parents, early childhood practitioners, and students. It transforms how we understand the relationship between young children and moving image media, offering a refreshing and informed alternative to screen-use guidelines.

Cary Bazalgette is an Honorary Research Associate at UCL Institute of Education, within the Department of Culture, Communication and Media. She specialises in how people learn to understand moving image media. After teaching in London schools, she worked at the British Film Institute from 1979 to 2007, including eight years as Head of Education. Her primary focus has been on developing good practices in media education and advocating for its importance as an essential entitlement for all learners. Currently, her research focuses on how children begin learning about moving image media before age three. Cary draws on her 35 years of experience in education about moving image media, as well as her personal experiences as a parent and grandparent. For more information, visit www.carybazalgette.net.

Beyond Screen Time Guilt

The Role of TV and Video in Early Child Development

Cary Bazalgette

Routledge
Taylor & Francis Group
LONDON AND NEW YORK

Designed cover image: Getty images

First published 2027
by Routledge
4 Park Square, Milton Park, Abingdon, Oxon OX14 4RN

and by Routledge
605 Third Avenue, New York, NY 10158

Routledge is an imprint of the Taylor & Francis Group, an informa business

British Library Cataloguing-in-Publication Data
A catalogue record for this book is available from the British Library

ISBN: 9781041266297 (hbk)
ISBN: 9781041266280 (pbk)
ISBN: 9781003751236 (ebk)

DOI: 10.4324/9781003751236

Typeset in Sabon
by Newgen Publishing UK

This book is dedicated to my grandchildren:
Morgan, Connie, and Alfie

Contents

Figures

Acknowledgements

I first became curious about children's TV-watching in the 1970s, hurrying back from the Coram Centre nursery with my children, Ben and Phoebe, and getting home in time to watch *Play School*. Later, when my husband Terry Staples programmed weekly film screenings for children at the National Film Theatre, and ran the short-lived Children's London Film Festival, I was able to listen and observe as children reacted to a historically and internationally diverse range of feature films. The pupils at Greenwich Park School in the 1960s, and at Holloway School in the 1970s, boosted my confidence about showing film extracts in the classroom. My British Film Institute (BFI) colleagues David Lusted, Jim Cook, Philip Simpson, and Manuel Alvarado extended my education about film, and my interest in younger children's understanding of moving image media was fostered by Ken Fox, Yvonne Davies, Jackie Marsh, Maire Messenger Davies, and Lydia Plowman. John Potter, Rosie Flewitt, and Liz Brooker supervised my PhD research; Julian Sefton-Green and David Buckingham provided helpful comments and advice in the book-writing process. My grandchildren Morgan, Alfie, and Connie have generously allowed me to observe them and write about them and, in the twins' case, to include photos of them as toddlers. Barry Ecuyer's witty and apposite drawings provide an important dimension of the book. Thanks to Sophie and Alex Charlton-Graham, for permission to use the pictures of Evie, and likewise to Yonas Tamene for the picture of Sunu. Pablo Griffiths provided vital technological advice and help with the documents and images. But it's my partner David Mitchell who has been closest to the process of writing this book; I couldn't have done it without his sensible corrections, thought-provoking comments, and loving patience.

Introduction

In 2005, 1500 UK parents answered a survey about their children's TV-viewing: 50% said that their babies had started watching it by the time they were three months old (Marsh et al., 2005). A more recent study, now that we've got mobile phones, tablets, and YouTube Kids, has found that 75% of UK babies are established viewers of TV and video on demand (VOD) by the time they're 12 months old, not only at home but also on phones or tablets in their prams and buggies, as can often be seen in supermarkets, cafes, and on public transport. But if you search online for answers to a question such as "is TV bad for babies?" you will get dozens of warnings, from sources that seem to be authoritative, about the supposedly terrible effects of early viewing on key aspects of development: brain growth, speech, social skills, and sleep time can all suffer, they say. And yet, a recent UK Department of Health review of child health showed that between 2024 and 2025, 81.4% of UK two-year-olds reached the expected levels of development in all five of the key domains that the review measures: communication skills, gross and fine motor skills, problem solving, and personal social skills. This was a slightly higher percentage than in their previous report, and part of an ongoing trend (*Child Development Outcomes 2024-2025: statistical commentary*, 2025).

I think that apparently simple questions like "what's good (or bad) for babies" never have simple answers, unless they are to do with obvious things like real physical safety and health. In this book, I take a completely different line from the usual arguments and dire warnings about 0–3-year-olds' relationships with "screens." It's based on my own parenting experience, my professional life as an educator, extensive reading, discussions with lots of parents and grandparents, and visits to social media. It draws on my own doctoral research, in which I didn't ask "bad or good?" questions but did very close observation of my twin grandchildren's viewing behaviour over a 20-month period, starting when they were 17 months old. Very few other researchers have done studies like this. I videoed the children while they watched and re-watched short films, episodes from their favourite TV series, and a few feature films. I wanted to catch their reactions to stories that they

DOI: 10.4324/9781003751236-1

already knew and liked, and to stories that I thought they would like. And I used video so that I could take time to look carefully at tiny features of their behaviour as they watched. I have included several images of the twins in this book because I know, from discussions with other parents and grandparents, as well as from my research reading, that they were typical toddlers.

Unlike most of the academics who claim that TV damages children's mental and physical health, I've worked as a media educator, teaching about the techniques that are used in film and TV to create meaning, and finding out the extent to which most children understand them. This was the basis of my research: I was able to interpret the children's viewing behaviour and responses, not only as a grandparent who knew them well, but also in relation to close analyses of the material they were watching at the time: the techniques of storytelling and presentation as well as the content. Everyone who enjoys viewing TV or film has had to learn to understand these techniques but hardly anyone remembers that, so most people don't feel that they have much technical knowledge about "film language." In Chapter 3 of this book, I describe the common techniques that film-makers use: you may not know what they're called, but you are certainly able to understand them. When you were a baby, you might have found them hard to follow at first, but that wouldn't have put you off watching and re-watching TV programmes or films.

I've written this book for two reasons. Firstly, because I think that 0–3-year-olds' intense drive to learn and explore TV and film needs to be recognised and studied. Secondly, because I believe that the moving image media that are viewed by babies and toddlers deserve serious attention. Children have the right to encounter, learn to understand and enjoy a wide range of story-telling styles in these media. They're an important part of most people's cultural experiences, and of many people's lives. As children grow older, parents and teachers can help and encourage them to develop the skills they'll need to make their own informed decisions about what kinds of media material they think are worthwhile, as well as to identify, challenge, and reject moving image material on TV and online that is deliberately misleading or exploitative. This argument does not affect the fact that books and print media are obviously more important – and of course more physically durable and accessible – than the moving image.

Am I arguing that babies and toddlers can be left to watch TV or videos for hours on end? Of course not: they shouldn't be left to do anything for hours on end! They need as much attention, variety, and activity as possible. But parenting is stressful enough without being made to feel guilty about something that obviously fascinates children, as well as being an important part of our culture, for all age-groups. If you are anxious about parents initiating conversations about whether or not 0–3s ought to see TV programmes or other moving image media, whether on TV or on mobile devices, this book will help you explore the issues with them. And if you are involved as a professional in discussions about whether 0–3s should be viewing these media at all, this book will at least give you more evidence about how they view than you're likely to get online, so that you can make informed contributions.

I hope that this book will encourage you to recognise and think about the extraordinary, self-driven learning that enables babies and toddlers to understand this complicated and important cultural form. The practical implications for managing their moving image experiences will then be up to you.

References

Child Development Outcomes 2024-2025: Statistical commentary. (2025). London: Department of Health and Social Care. Retrieved from www.gov.uk/government/statistics/child-development-outcomes-at-2-to-2-and-a-half-years-april-2023-to-march-2024-annual-2023-to-2024/child-development-outcomes-at-2-to-2-and-a-half-years-2023-to-2024-statistical-commentary

Marsh, J., Brooks, G., Hughes, J., Ritchie, L., Roberts, S., & Wright, K. (2005). *Digital Beginnings: Young children's use of popular culture, media and new technologies*. Retrieved from Sheffield: www.researchgate.net/publication/265183910_Digital_beginnings_Young_children%27s_use_of_popular_culture_media_and_new_technologies (accessed 08-11-2021)

Chapter 1

What "screen time" really involves

Dad's in a hurry. Four-month-old Baby Sunu has been quite a handful this evening – Mum is busy, and he's late getting to work. Using a familiar trick so that he can finish his dinner, he's popped Sunu on his lap and put his phone on a stool close by, so that she can watch an episode of *Cocomelon*.

In Figure 1.1, the phone screen that Sunu is watching shows a close-up of a face, with the very big eyes which are typical of this series (and of many other TV programmes for babies and toddlers) and which seem to be focused on something off-screen. The chances are that the next shot will show what that character is looking at, though Sunu may not yet be very skilful in following another person's gaze in real life, in which case she won't be anticipating the next shot (more about "point-of-view shots" in Chapter 3). Nevertheless, eyes are very important for babies in their growing relationships with other people. The makers of *Cocomelon*, and of many other "baby TV" series, are well aware of this, which is why the characters' eyes in most series are shown as proportionately much bigger than real human or animal eyes (more about the significance of eye contact, and its eventual relationship to humans' development of language, in Chapter 4).

Of course, you don't know Sunu, but you may still notice that her head is raised in order to see the screen properly: that takes a bit of effort for a baby lying on her tummy, whose head, at only four months, is much bigger than an older child's in proportion to her body. And from what we can see of her face, she's looking very serious. We can only see her right eye: it's wide open and intent. Maybe she is also frowning a bit: because babies and toddlers have such plump faces, it's hard to tell when they are frowning, and here we can only see one side of her face anyway. Look at her hands: her right hand is clenched, perhaps grasping the edge of her blanket, while her left hand is extended, the fingers tightly pinched together, with the thumb tucked in. Hand positions are a good indicator of her level of bodily tension: she's very alert at the moment. We can't easily see her mouth, which is also a good indicator, but it does seem to be closed, which also indicates attentiveness. So, although she's keeping still, and we have quite a limited view of her, it looks as though Sunu is investing a lot of energy in her TV-viewing.[1]

DOI: 10.4324/9781003751236-2

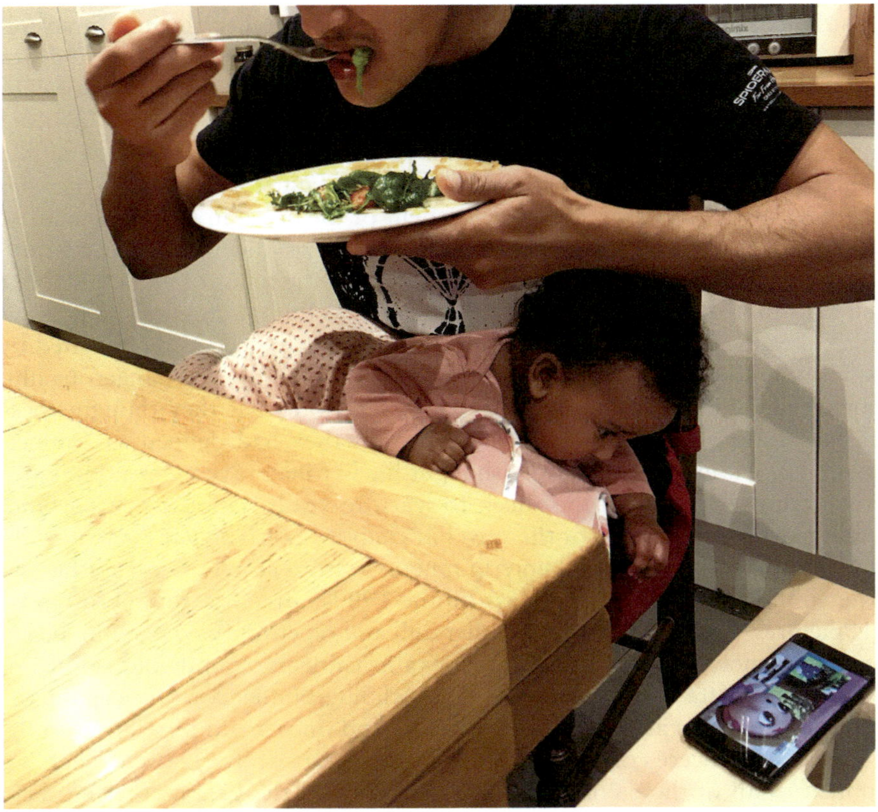

Figure 1.1 Dad and Sunu. Photo: Cary Bazalgette.

One of the mothers I met during my PhD research told me early in an interview that her two-year-old son just stared at TV "like a zombie." About half an hour later, after she'd told me a lot more about his viewing habits, I asked whether she had really meant the "zombie" comparison, and whether being quiet and still could be interpreted differently. She eagerly retracted the "zombie" word, insisting that her son did concentrate closely and she was proud of how he made a real effort to understand what he was watching. She admitted that she wasn't sure why she'd said "zombie," though I suspect it was because at that stage of the interview I hadn't yet told her about my motivations for doing the research, and she had assumed that I would be going along with the popular idea that watching TV doesn't demand much effort.

It does seem as though expressions such as "passive viewing" or "couch potato" have become almost default terms in conversations about TV viewing, even in wry admissions such as "I was so knackered yesterday! When

I got home, I just turned into a couch potato and watched the first three episodes of that new thing on Netflix." In Chapter 2, I note the widespread use of terms such as "exposure," "passive viewing," and "use" to characterise TV-viewing by babies and toddlers, all of which imply that no effort is involved in watching TV. But the passivity idea is probably linked to the longstanding belief that uneducated audiences will always be vulnerable to ill-effects from any new leisure medium. The development of the novel in the 18th century, music hall in the 19th century, cinema and television in the 20th century, and "screens" in the 21st century, have all been the focus of anxieties about the risks that they were assumed to present to certain sectors of the population. In each case, these assumptions have been expressed and circulated by people who considered themselves competent to identify the dangerous illusions, timewasting fantasies, and unruly behaviour that they thought these media would encourage in the social groups they had defined as "vulnerable." For example, novels were thought likely to deprave women (and also any servants who'd had the cheek to learn to read): Jane Austen parodies posh male dismissiveness of the novel in chapter 1 of *Northanger Abbey*. In the 19th century, music hall entertainments were accused of corrupting and over-stimulating the working class. In the 1900s, attention shifted to "moving pictures" when that initially rather dull and repetitive new medium began to develop new techniques (editing, movable cameras, sound, and colour) to tell stories, create star performers, and reach huge audiences. Once again, the same assumptions about risks were made, and once again in relation to the audiences that were considered "vulnerable" – especially children. There's a subtext to all of these comments, I think: it's that the people uttering them are really thinking "these people shouldn't be wasting time with this sort of stuff: they should be doing their jobs/doing their homework/getting on with something useful."

The kind of audiences that were considered vulnerable to bad influences from popular entertainment forms increased enormously in the 20th century, when the scale, nature, and accessibility of popular entertainment began to expand. The concept of a "mass audience" (i.e. large, dispersed, passive, and disdained by posher people) began to be commonplace. In the 1920s, the concept of a large and vulnerable audience began to include children; by the 1950s, children, and especially teenagers, were increasingly the centre of concern. The focus of anxieties about how new media and allegedly "cheap content" might negatively affect them broadened to include cinema, television, comics, video, and, by the beginning of the 21st century, video games, the internet, and then social media. An increasing number of academic research projects tried to identify whether there really are risks involved in reading horror comics or watching violent TV programmes, and what might be the longer-term outcomes of these activities for children and teenagers. The more recent concerns about the addictiveness of social media and, in particular, the "digital sexual abuse" apps that became available in 2025 on Elon Musk's Grok AI tool, making it possible to create pornographic images from any photo of a person – child or adult – are of a different order, inviting users to collaborate in abuse, so generating widespread public disgust and immediate calls for bans. But in this book I am focusing only on moving image media.

There are two problems with basing academic research on children's viewing behaviour and the question of whether or not the enjoyment of cultural material such as TV programmes carries risks, especially long-term ones. Firstly, it is that the terms of the inquiry tend to be focused on a search for effects, and to spend little or no time on the viewing process itself or on what is actually watched. Secondly, viewing is usually referred to in the research literature as either "consumption" or "exposure": both terms imply that there is little effort on the part of the viewers. "Consumption" invokes images of gobbling up and swallowing, and is not how most of us describe our cultural activities. Do you "consume" pictures in a photo album, music on your headphones, or a story in a novel? Are you "exposed" to poetry or concerts? It seems to betray a hidden prejudice against audiences for newer media: a belief that certain kinds of people will just passively gulp in "the latest" in images, stories, ideas, and information that are presented to them; they don't have any critical skills for judging their value (or lack of it); they won't learn anything from them but will nevertheless develop an appetite for more. When the same kinds of judgements are made about babies and children, they are motivated by assumptions about vulnerability and innocence, more rarely by condescension. But "exposure" usually implies some sort of risk, whether from something everyday like sunshine, or from something highly dangerous: nuclear fallout, for example. And when used in relation to babies, it may remind us of the practice in some ancient cultures for getting rid of unwanted babies by leaving them "exposed" in some desolate place to die. Both terms imply that television viewing just means passively absorbing a mass of essentially similar stuff. Few researchers have acknowledged the fact that is probably obvious to the rest of us: that if there are any "effects" from television viewing, they must depend on what kinds of programme are watched. Frazer was one – very early, and widely ignored – exception (Frazer, 1981).

In fact, there isn't really a word that covers the combination of skills that people use when they watch a TV programme or a cinema film – though some people do use "reading." A range of elements all contribute to how we interpret their meaning: framing, movement, colour, lighting, perspective, focus, spoken words, actions, facial expressions, settings, costume are features of the filming process; along with the editing techniques that follow (and that I describe in Chapter 3), they all contribute to the processes of storytelling. The stories themselves lean heavily on the themes and conventions of the cultures in which they are made, so babies and toddlers are learning about these from the material they watch as well as from the cultures in which they themselves have been born into (more about cultures and social viewing in Chapter 9, and in Chapter 10, there's a comparison between two currently popular series for children that handle cultural conventions very differently). But to start with, they have to learn how to "read" the media that they watch.

Moving image productions for children are made in one or other (and sometimes more than one!) of the many animation formats and technologies that are now available; Wikipedia will tell you more about these than you may want to bother remembering. I shall not attempt to list or define them here (there's more detail in Chapter 3 about filming and editing): the basic point is that all these elements are, to some degree, meaningful. They affect, and sometimes determine, how we interpret and emotionally respond to what we see and hear. I haven't been able to find a suitable term for referring to the process of understanding moving image media. Some people (including me) have used "reading" to refer to that, but it doesn't seem right to me any longer. So now I just tend to rely on "viewing" rather than "watching," because I think that may imply a rather more active process.

In Figure 1.1, it is obvious that at four months, Sunu must have been able to see things that were significant for her, and that she was concentrating very hard as she viewed. *Cocomelon* characters always have huge heads and enormous eyes, as do many other "baby TV" programmes: we know that faces are extremely important, especially to babies. We also know that babies quickly become responsive to changes of expression: smiles, raised eyebrows, widened eyes, and (less often, we hope) frowns and pursed lips. New-borns watch faces closely as they build relationships with the people around them, soon starting to recognise facial expressions and to interpret emotions: faces are meaningful! Learning to understand them can be exciting and satisfying. Viewing episodes from a TV series enables babies and toddlers to become familiar with its conventions and style. They will gradually start to look at other things within the story: people and/or objects that may either be in the frame, or are soon revealed; actions, the things that motivate them, and their consequences (more about this in Chapter 5). Viewing episodes repeatedly underpins and starts to extend their interpretive skills.

From their first contacts with TV, babies and toddlers gradually get to understand the techniques of story-telling in moving images. They start to follow – and probably soon anticipate – actions and consequences. So, crucially, they are starting to learn how to make sense of this fascinating medium. This is the other central point of my argument in this book: that in their first three years of life, children who view TV and film *must be learning how to understand them.* They do this voluntarily, eagerly, and intensively, using repeat viewing to consolidate their learning. And as what they view is not all the same, each new programme or series that they encounter presents them with new learning: a challenge that they meet with the kind of dedicated attention that Figure 1.1 illustrates. In Chapter 3, I explain this learning in more detail; in Chapter 9, I compare two well-known but contrasting TV series for babies and toddlers, identifying some of the learning challenges that they may present; in Chapter 11, I describe why and how children move on from one favourite programme or series to another. My starting-point is radically different from almost all of the other research that has investigated little children and moving image media, where the focus is too often on whether children gain "educationally relevant" information and knowledge (usually words, colours, numbers, and letters) *from* these media. There are of course TV series that set out to do that (e.g. *Sesame Street*) but my argument in this book is that learning *how stories are told*, learning *how to recognise* different kinds of story – for example, those that are meant to be funny – is also to contribute to the important skills and knowledge about social environments and established behaviours that babies and toddlers are learning about in daily life at the same time. The simplest proof that such learning must happen is that a one-year-old can't follow a 90-minute feature film for child audiences, but many three-year-olds can, and five-year-olds certainly do.

When it comes to considering how very young children understand and respond to TV programmes and films, anyone faces problems in trying to interpret what they are actually doing. Laughter, excitement, fear, and sadness can usually be identified quite easily, but if a child who doesn't have much language yet seems intent on, or even fascinated by, what they are viewing, how can one tell what it is that interests them and what they make of it? Obviously, it helps if one knows the child and is already used to noticing what kinds of things they're currently intrigued by, so parents are best-placed to interpret their child's viewing behaviour. But – let's be honest – parents often need to take advantage of their child's attentiveness to a TV programme if it's finally given them time to take a shower or make the dinner, so they may not have extended opportunities to watch what their child is doing when she is viewing TV. She is likely to have periods of close concentration (like Sunu's) in which her posture and expressions may not change much, but it takes very close observation – perhaps even using video, as I did – if one is to spot minute details like a frown, or the tiny rim of tears round her eyes when something has made her feel sad. She may also have clenched hands, or even just a very still posture, perhaps supported by holding on to a nearby bit of furniture. I saw a lot of this kind of thing during my PhD research, and I did have to use video (unobtrusively caught on my mobile phone) and study it closely afterwards to realise how frequent and extensive it was.

It can often be grandparents (like me) who are best-placed to observe a child's viewing behaviour. We've "seen it all before" and we're less likely to be anxious about such things as the child's pace of development, although in some families it's the grandparents who most disapprove of TV-watching.

But both parents and grandparents are potentially better at interpreting a child's viewing behaviour than an academic researcher who may visit for a couple of hours a week at most. Many researchers attempt to observe the behaviour of children in a university "lab," which may be organised to look like an "ordinary living room," as the research reports often claim (see also Chapter 2, and the Moonbug research described in Chapter 4). Some have used video material specially made to test children's ability to remember or learn from what they see, which inevitably has none of the expensive features of commercial TV, such as colour, 3D figures, depth of field, music, and so on, and is consequently unlikely to hold a child's attention for long, but that hasn't stopped researchers claiming it as proof that children "can't learn from video" (see my discussion of the "video deficit effect" in Chapter 2).

Another pitfall that can be hard to avoid, if one doesn't know a child really well, is the temptation to make assumptions about what they are doing, based on stereotypical notions associated with "what little children are like." For example, the common phenomenon of a toddler touching the TV screen is often interpreted as them thinking that something on the screen is actually real, based on the conventional idea that little children are naïve and innocent, and don't understand that the things on the screen aren't really "there" (I discuss this in Chapter 8). We are of course bound to view our children tenderly and to be aware that there are many things they don't yet know – from some of which they may need to be protected. But we do also know what voracious explorers they are, once they are mobile, and it won't hurt to recognise this as necessary (more on this in Chapter 4) though obviously we still have to interfere in some of their experiments, such as trying to play with the knife drawer or to post your debit card through a gap in the floorboards.

This book, then, is not about the effects of viewing moving image media, apart from enjoyment, and the short-term reactions of fear, sadness, and laughter. I'm not claiming that there aren't any effects, but whatever they are, they're extremely various and dependent upon many other factors. The claims that you can find online, assembled by a search engine's AI in response to a question about the effects of TV on young children – for example, that it "can hinder their development by delaying language skills, impacting their attention span, reducing physical activity, potentially disrupting sleep patterns ... taking away from crucial real-life learning experiences with caregivers and their environment" are not about TV itself, but about poor parenting practices that could be associated with TV-viewing for some children (and see Chapter 2). If these effects really were to occur in all the 75% of babies who start watching TV in their first year (according to the research finding that I quote in the "Introduction" chapter of this book), the consequent social, health, and even economic problems would be enormous!

In relation to claims that TV-watching has long-term effects such as low achievement in school (Zimmerman & Christakis, 2005), it's important to note that in some circumstances parents have little choice but to depend on a TV set or an iPhone to keep their child occupied, and that unfortunately there are children who are neglected, ignored, and lacking in other resources, for whom TV may be the only thing available to keep them occupied. In such situations, it's obvious that it's the lack of other stimulation that's the problem, and perhaps the TV might be, in some cases, better than nothing. Until recently, a great deal of the research on "TV effects" failed to find out about family circumstances, but this has recently begun to change, as I explain in Chapter 2.

My arguments in this book are based on the fact that all moving image media (TV, film, VOD) are *cultural forms*: they include a wide range of genres (even, though to a lesser extent, within TV for 0–3s); they offer us many different kinds of experience; and they continue to develop and change. People who enjoy them differ enormously in what they like to view, react to, comment on, and discuss with their friends and/or within their families. Some people view a lot and some only view a little – or none. Increasingly, TV may not be viewed in the living room, but on mobile devices, though many families still enjoy getting together to view a current favourite, whether that's drama, sport, comedy, documentary, or news (and those of us who view *Gogglebox* on UK Channel 4 enjoy seeing them enjoy it). Increasingly, people download material from YouTube, Netflix, and other online sources (that's VOD or "video on demand"), whether for individual or shared viewing. An enormous part of what babies and toddlers have to learn to understand is the culture into which they have been born. Everything around them is part of that culture – talk, food, clothes, pictures, furniture, toys, books, music – and, of course, VOD, and television.

Culture is a specifically human phenomenon. Michael Tomasello argues that "Humans are able to coordinate with others, in a way that other primates seemingly are not, to form a "we" that acts as a kind of plural agent to create everything from a collaborative hunting party to a cultural institution" (Tomasello, 2014).

The reason he includes a "hunting party" relates to his belief that as prehumans became bipedal, they had to develop ways of communicating to each other – to start with, by hand gestures and eye direction; later with sounds – especially during the tense, vital, and collaborative process of stalking prey, but also while they were foraging for fruit or nuts – and that vocal communications in some form are highly likely to have started developing in those contexts and, over thousands of years, to become shareable, learnable, complex languages. In Chapter 5, I discuss further the question of how human language may have developed, and with it all the shared information, ideas, and stories that are the foundation of human cultures. And Chapter 9 is about how learning to understand the TV and film material that their families like to view, and about starting to understand and join in with others' responses, can be important parts of how children become part of their families' shared cultures.

My primary aims in this book are, firstly, to argue for little children's right to watch and learn to understand the moving image material that they find fascinating and enjoyable, to share that pleasure with their families, and to go on discovering different styles and types of moving image media. Much later – and beyond the scope of this book – they should be helped to develop the critical skills that will enable them to decide what they think is worth watching and, in the case of the many forms of moving image-based information they will encounter, what to believe. My second aim is to offer you insights and ideas that may help alert you to what's going on in the early stages of a child's learning about moving image media, to help you recognise, appreciate, and encourage their efforts and, if you are an Early Years practitioner, to share these insights and ideas with parents.

TAKEAWAYS

Talking with families

Any discussion with parents about their child's TV- and/or video-watching *should be initiated by them*, and conducted tactfully, until it is clear what their attitudes and practices are. If you initiate the conversation, they are likely to worry that you're going to tell them that their child/ren shouldn't watch TV. If they are adamant about TV having bad effects on children and either limit or ban viewing, don't try to contradict or argue with them. But if they admit (maybe nervously!) that their child does enjoy some – or even a lot – of TV and VOD, they may be happy to tell you what s/he enjoys, and maybe recount stories of viewing occasions when they were scared or amused.

Observation

If you have an opportunity (which may well be brief, and probably rare) to observe a child viewing a programme on TV or a video on a smartphone or tablet, you might try to note their behaviour, for example, level of attention, expression, posture, reactions. Children of 2+ might be responsive to questions about straightforward things such as a character's name, why a character is doing something noticeable, and so on. The aim of such questioning would be to gain a sense of how well they understand what they are viewing, whether they enjoy it, and if so, what bits they especially like. If they don't like it that much, you could try to find out whether there is a specific thing, character, or moment that is off-putting or maybe even scary (see Chapter 7 for discussion of fears).

Further reading

Arnold, C. (2021). *Observing Gabby*. Open University Press. Study by a grandmother and Early Years expert, of her grandchild from 0 to 6 years: a fine example of close observation of a very young child.

Note

1 Here and throughout the book I'll be using the term "TV" that would include both streamed and broadcast TV episodes, and will also refer to video on demand (VOD) which can be watched individually on mobile devices, or on TV screens.

References

Frazer, C. F. (1981). The social character of children's television viewing. *Communication Research, 8*(3), 307–322.

Tomasello, M. (2014). *A natural history of human thinking*. Cambridge, Mass.: Harvard University Press.

Zimmerman, F. J., & Christakis, D. A. (2005). Children's television viewing and cognitive outcomes. *Archives of Pediatrics & Adolescent Medicine, 159*.

Chapter 2

What "screen time" research has – and hasn't – told us

Research that has looked for evidence about how TV-watching may affect babies' and toddlers' development is often invoked in discussions about childcare, usually on the basis of a general awareness that there has been such research and it has proved that such young children should have little or no "screen time." There has indeed been a great deal of such research, especially studies looking for what were assumed to be the risks of TV-watching for babies and toddlers. This has now begun to change, as I shall show in this chapter. Although warnings about the supposed negative effects of TV-watching by 0–3s are still widespread, I have seen a gradual change in the tone of the warnings that usually follow any online search for answers to a question such as "is TV bad for babies?." The first three of the 15,200 results I got from asking Google that on March 12, 2026, were slightly more nuanced than those I'd got from a similar search three months before. There are still plenty of scary warnings about the alleged effects of TV-watching, attributed to "research," though online search results rarely provide sources. Effects on babies' brain development, behaviour, learning, and life-chances are still cited, together with the assumption that TV is always "passively watched." But online searches do now turn up some acknowledgements of the pleasures of TV and VOD, pressures on parents, and even the possibilities of learning from TV.

These changes may be reflecting the modifications that the influential American Association of Pediatrics (AAP) have started to make to their "screen time" advice. They did finally realise that most of the research they had drawn on to support their original rules and warnings about the supposed dire effects of TV-watching on babies' brain development and later school performance was badly designed and unreliable. Announcing this in 2016, they said that "the relationship between time spent on screen media and negative health and wellbeing outcomes is complex and depends on many factors" and admitted that "the research guiding our understanding of the impact of screen media on health and wellbeing is further complicated by inconsistent or inaccurate research measures." This change of policy was good news for those of us who had been criticising it for several years,

DOI: 10.4324/9781003751236-3

although many people have already internalised the old advice and think they know that "All TV is bad for babies and toddlers." The AAP's updated summary of their screen time guidelines for children and teens is available online at www.aap.org/en/patient-care/media-and-children/center-of-excellence-on-social-media-and-youth-mental-health/qa-portal/qa-portal-library/qa-portal-library-questions/screen-time-guidelines/.

However, the data that I quoted in the "Introduction" do indicate that most parents have never stuck to the old advice anyway, and that the babies and toddlers who were "exposed" to the "effects" of TV can't have been adversely affected. That is indicated by the UK's Department of Health comments, which said in 2025 that the percentage of 2-year-olds reaching top levels of the Department's five standard measures of development had been increasing for the previous five years "for all domains apart from communication skills, which is stable" (*Child Development Outcomes 2024-2025: statistical commentary*, 2025). That is despite all the TV-viewing most babies had been doing: 75% of them had probably been viewing since they were less than 12 months old (Barber et al., 2017).

Although the unproven claim that TV can damage babies' brains is still included in online search results, much of the advice does now show a shift towards "good parenting," at least in the case of advice for parents of babies. The "screen time" advice gets more confusing when older children are included. The AAP's instructions (as of February 2026) have moved "beyond simple time limits to focus on quality, context and conversation" and draw upon research at the Children's Hospital of Orange County (https://health.choc.org/updated-aap-recommendations-for-screen-time/). They stress that "screen time itself isn't the enemy," prioritising quality, context, and conversation over strict time limits, although they do still rule on "no screens before 18 months and one hour of high-quality content daily for age 2–5."

On March 27, 2026, the UK Government issued new guidance on "screen use by children under five," which was close to the AAP's latest pronouncements, although with one key change "Children under the age of five should be limited to one hour of screen time a day, while under-twos should not be watching screens alone" – thus showing a marked and important shift towards "good parenting" and away from time-based instructions. The guidance was based on a review by ten senior academic researchers, commissioned jointly by the Department for Education and the Department of Health and Social Care, and established as the Early Years Screen Time Advisory Group in January 2026 (EYSTAG, 2026). They selected 63 "systematic reviews" for close analysis from a long list of 632 reviews of research on small children's engagements with screen media, and also received 132 responses to their call for evidence on February 2, 2026. Their remit involved a continued use of the "screen time" label, despite its obvious potential for confusion, given the enormous expansion of different kinds of screen-based devices in this century. However, in the context of quickly understandable slogans and rulings, it has become the best option, although some paranoid minorities might leap to the conclusion that the guidance wasn't just about TV and VOD but was also trying to stop babies using social media. The UK's review was commissioned soon after the Australian government's ban on social media accounts for under 16s (widely reported, however, as "screen use"), which took effect on December 10, 2025, and was widely debated.

For the higher age-groups, much of the older, scarier advice remains. There can be many good reasons for not watching TV during meals, such as missing out on social interaction, but the online search I used only turned up "childhood obesity," adding the vague, and almost certainly unprovable (hence the get-out word "can") statement that "excessive screen time can also be linked to sleep disturbances and other issues later in life." The search results also included the hackneyed phrase "passive screen time" (which, as you will see in later chapters – if you don't know it already – practically never applies to real toddlers) as something that will lead to "atypical sensory behaviors and may impact social-emotional development." These are quasi-scientific terms designed to frighten non-academic parents, also used in other warnings, such as "Delayed language development" and "Increased sedentary time." And the newly fashionable use of "impact" as a verb is obviously more alarming than "affect," even if many people may not be sure what "social-emotional" means.

Much of the research that these "effects" claims are based on has been done in the USA, unsurprisingly, since it has been the AAP's statements that have dominated most of the advice. It took the AAP until 2016 to admit that the research they had used was not fit for purpose, although even in the 1990s, there had been critics who found fault with it. For example, the late Colwyn Trevarthen, Professor of child Psychology and Psychobiology at the University of Edinburgh, made this comment in 1998, suggesting that notions of emotional security and economically useful independent thinking might be dominating, and perhaps narrowing, the US researchers' concerns:

> The psychology textbooks that our students read, most from the USA, are lively and full of facts, but they give a strange account of the forces that lead a child to become a citizen. Apparently, the two main tasks are to construct an emotionally secure self-image and then to acquire independent and rational thinking that can be put to effect in economically useful work.
>
> (Trevarthen, 1998)

Trevarthen's focus in his book chapter was, as mine is, on the importance of culture, even in the earliest stages of children's lives. So he was understandably concerned by the pre-eminence that American academics seemed to give to more instrumental, goal-driven priorities in child-rearing, and forgetting other values that cultural experiences can help to generate, such as empathy and imagination. I recalled this comment as I read papers on children and TV published after 2000, when concerns were becoming focused on "screen time" and, a bit later, on "digital exposure," and when it was recognised that increasing numbers of babies and toddlers (like the rest of us) are accessing visual material on mobile devices as well as on TV sets. I was particularly intrigued by the language used in these papers. I discuss researchers' use of "exposed" in Chapter 1. These terms imply that children do not choose to watch specific programmes or series, or even express any preferences about what they want to see, but are either just positioned in front of screens, whatever they may happen to be showing, or merely stick with whatever comes up when they switch on a device, with the added implication that whatever does come up is not going to be of much value, at least in terms of career-oriented priorities, and might even be dangerous. Occasionally, the word "use" occurs instead, but without any indication of what the screens might be used for: sometimes expanded into "addictive use," "problematic use," "media use habits," "technology use," etc. Again, "use" is an implicitly negative term, given that it is always used in discussions of drug addiction. So both "exposure" and "use" imply that no process of interpretation is involved in watching moving image media: that viewers just passively "consume" it. In Chapter 6, I discuss the tendency for parents (and grandparents, and anyone else involved) to use these terms when discussing "screen time."

Many researchers on children and TV were preoccupied with what they thought "screen time" is for. If it is going to be allowed at all, it should be for learning, in their opinion. This is still an important principle for many academics in this field, and is another reason why Trevarthen's comments came to mind when I was reading them. The "learning" that some academics still look for is not the "learning about" that I am focusing upon in this book, but "learning from": that is, acquiring knowledge of words, colours, and numbers to start with, and then their written forms, and going on to facts about the world: places, things, activities, rules, etc.; in other words, learning that's going to be useful, and may help children to "get ahead" when they start school.

There are a few academics who recognise that 0–3s don't understand TV or video the first time they see it. Daniel Anderson has been writing about this for many years and has used techniques of eye-tracking to analyse how toddlers react to what they are watching. He acknowledges that moving image media use editing to construct meanings, and that this "montage" (as he calls it) isn't immediately understood by novice viewers. But I find his descriptions of editing techniques strangely impersonal, in that they take no account of the instinctive behaviour that they relate to, or to the emotional effects that they can have (Anderson & Kirkorian, 2018): essentially, he does not seem to consider TV as a cultural form. Back in 1979, Anderson also originated the weird "attentional inertia" theory (essentially, "the more they watch, the more they watch"), and the "video deficit theory" which I discuss later in this chapter (Anderson et al., 1979). Some interesting studies have focused on aspects of children's developing understanding of television, linked to specific features or techniques (Calvert, 1988; Lowe & Durkin, 1999; Wass & Smiht, 2015), but they tend to use experimental techniques or short-term studies, rather than examining their longer-term learning about the medium.

Obviously, it's important for children to learn things from their families and maybe also from their media experiences, but there is a lot more that they have to learn about media as well: about how they tell stories and communicate meanings, that will become vital later in life if they ever want to challenge the truth of moving image communications. I explain more about this in the following chapters, as well as describing babies and toddlers' responses to the varied array of material that is created to appeal to their emotions and to help develop their sense of humour, while at the same time developing their skills in understanding stories, characters, and genres. The "learning from" principle ignores the features that really attract babies and children to these media in the first place, such as movement, colour, faces, music, and voices – features that they are already recognising and learning to interpret in daily life – and from which they will eventually learn how to follow a story, understand characters' motivations and states of mind, develop expectations, and, eventually, become able to recognise genres and make informed choices about what they do and don't like. This is *cultural learning*: as I argued in Chapter 1, it supports, extends, and contributes to the learning that babies are doing all the time anyway, as part of the communities they've been born into.

The universal beginnings of this learning are signalled when a baby becomes able, at six weeks old or so, to respond with a smile when someone smiles at them; by laughing when they are aged three or four months; at around nine months being able to follow someone else's gaze, and soon after that by starting to talk. All these and many other things that parents eagerly wait for are crucial moments in becoming part of any human community: subtle indicators of emotional states and non-verbal ways of expressing feelings through glances, expressions, gestures, and other body language. Inevitably, these indicators also feature in storytelling, whether in live social situations or in dramatic performances, dance, sport, or filmed narratives, from home videos to feature films, and of course in the animated or live action stories that babies may start watching on TV or on mobile devices, from three months old or even younger. Babies who don't watch these media aren't disadvantaged much (although later on they may feel a bit left out of some conversations and games when they get to nursery or reception class) but if they do watch them, they certainly will enjoy recognising the same facial expressions, body language, and hand gestures in both real-life and in fictions, eventually becoming able to anticipate the consequences in both contexts. At the same time, as well as becoming familiar with the culture of their family and community, they will be learning the techniques that are used to tell stories in moving image media, which I explain in Chapter 3.

A lot of research on children's "exposure" to "screens" has been done by academics who have never undertaken close analyses of moving image media, considered the diversity of content that babies and toddlers may be watching, or taken into account the widespread "re-viewing" phenomenon (discussed in Chapter 6). Some researchers have used techniques such as eye-tracking technology to find out whether babies can understand features of film editing (such as those I discuss in Chapter 3); Kirbas and Smith provide a review of such experiments (Kirbas & Smith, 2018). But experimental research on babies and toddlers has its limitations if it does not take into account their everyday-viewing behaviour over time: something that can only be properly established through extended observational studies. Of course, it is likely that a baby's first experience of a point-of-view shot or a jump cut (I explain these in Chapter 3) will be that they don't understand it, but the really interesting question is how and when they do learn it. If TV is just an incomprehensible sequence of images and sounds, why do they want to go on watching it? Why do they often want to watch the same things again and again, or express a particular preference for one series or show rather than another? Many of the studies cited by Kirbas and Smith identify techniques and conventions that babies or toddlers don't understand, but most of them are done in experimental settings. Viewing in familiar surroundings, in many cases with older siblings or with parents or grandparents, provides a context in which the younger children can soon become aware that what everyone else is viewing is meaningful and enjoyable. And in any case, even if their understanding is limited at first, they can understand enough to realise that there's more to discover. Some people get very concerned about little children not being able to understand something, characterising it as sad or at least unfortunate. I prefer to argue for the opposite: that it's intriguing, even exciting, to realise that there's more to discover: that it can motivate children to investigate further, and in the case of stories on TV or in books, to view or hear them again – maybe many times.

Research and debate about children and TV have often relied on characterising moving image media as "two-dimensional." This is a major over-simplification: presumably – and if so, naively – derived from the fact that the content is shown on flat screens. While it is obviously important for all children to experience real-life contacts and experience in the everyday three-dimensional world, moving image media devices such as depth of field, travelling shots, and point-of-view shots all not only provide representations of such a world but also emphasise them and invite curiosity. As we can see from the image at the beginning of Chapter 1, the off-screen gaze of the *Cocomelon* character provides an implied three-dimensionality to the scene and could provoke an older baby's curiosity: what are those huge eyes looking at? And my comparison of *Cocomelon* and *Bluey* episodes in Chapter 10 may help to explain how the sense of three-dimensional space can be created in a film.

My theory about what Sunu may be intrigued by is based on my assumption that the constant, highly emphasised presence of big eyes, that are seen in many "baby TV" programmes, must be contributing to, as well as building on, babies' growing awareness of eye direction and its importance in human culture. As Tomasello has argued, collective activities such as hunting by pre- and early humans, in which eye direction and expressions must have been vital, probably played a key part in the development of spoken language (see Chapters 1 and 5). Obviously, babies soon learn the significance of eye direction anyway, but even a mere corroboration of what is already a developing awareness will at least be pleasant and rewarding. It cannot be delaying the "brain development" that the researchers claim to be worrying about, and I wonder whether it could in fact be contributing to that development. Too many researchers are preoccupied with showing what babies and toddlers don't understand, and implying thereby that TV-viewing isn't appropriate for them.

One of the most long-standing and widely quoted theories in the research literature on children and moving image media is the "video deficit effect" (VDE), originally presented by Anderson and Pempek in the *American Behavioral Scientist* journal in 2005 (Anderson & Pempek, 2005). They used evidence from experimental observations to prove that very young children learn things like copying an action (hiding a toy, for example) more easily from a live demonstrator than they do from a video of someone demonstrating the same thing. On this basis, they propose that children learn better from real people than they do from video. My initial response, when I read their 2005 article, was that the video they used for the experiment must have been made to order by or for the academics, so it would inevitably have looked very different from the popular, high-budget children's television at the time – *Teletubbies*, for instance, or *Sesame Street*. To imagine that such a video could appear convincing or realistic to toddlers with many months of TV-watching experience seemed extraordinarily simplistic to me. The VDE has in fact come in for a lot of criticism over the years, recently, for example, from Sommer et al. in 2023, who point out that the increasing number of failures to repeat the 2005 observation "as children begin perceiving technology as relevant and meaningful in everyday life more and more" (Sommer et al., 2023). In 2011, Simcock et al. compared imitation from TV and picture books by 18- and 24-month-old children, finding that they could imitate from both, but more from TV (Simcock et al., 2011). And in 2008, Nielsen et al. demonstrated that a live demonstration by a "socially responsive" model would always be likely to appeal to children and make them likely to imitate them, but this didn't necessarily mean that video *per se* would always be in ineffective instructor (Nielsen et al., 2008).

Although none of us is two years old any more, we can still set up our own experiment to get some idea of the difference between video information and advice from a live person. Most of us have probably used one or more of the video demonstrations that come with some tricky piece of equipment. I was certainly a victim of VDE myself when I tried to use video instructions to find out how to fix the shower screen door: I ended up throwing the instruction kit across the room in a rage. Even instructional videos need some scripting and production skills!

However, we do all know that children can often copy things they are viewing, or that they have seen recently. So it seems that the VDE enthusiasts have never taken that into account. For example, the twins had a phase of running through the woods waving sticks and screaming "the big bad mouse is coming!" in imitation of the screen version of Julia Donaldson's novel *The Gruffalo's Child* (Magic Light Pictures, UK and Germany 2011), but that was driven by their enjoyment of a narrative trope, rather than by following instructions. However, they wouldn't stop when I asked them to. Perhaps acknowledging an "Instruction Deficit Effect" in toddlers would be helpful for parents struggling with "terrible twos" (see Chapter 4)?

But other researchers (Barr et al., 2007; Krcmar, 2010) and more recently (Kirbas & Smith, 2018) have repeated the VDE experiments, introducing different factors and showing them to children of different ages. They are also referred to in the EYSTAG report I discussed earlier. I suspect that the VDE claim is a helpful to those who want to argue that video (or TV) is inferior to real life. But the differences between cultural forms are never as simplistic as that. I suppose we could claim that *King Lear* or *Wuthering Heights* are not like real life and so we can't learn from them, but that would be to ignore their imaginative power and emotional impact. I would never claim that *Teletubbies* or *Bluey* have the same cultural value as the major classics, but they do nevertheless show recognisable human interactions and emotions, have engaging narrative structures, are enjoyable for many viewers, and could claim to be reinforcing children's appreciation of important things like kindness and friendship.

In any case, as I will show in later chapters, there is plenty of evidence that children do learn many things from TV, but they are things that are part of the knowledge that we all need in order to go on being able to interpret the stories and ideas that circulate in our culture: how to recognise the kind of story we are watching, or hearing, or reading. Is it meant to be funny? Or sad? Or scary? Is a character meant to be nice or nasty, or maybe just a bit suspicious? Is it a true story or a made-up one? Is this a programme for "children like me," or older people? Is it happening in a real place or an imaginary one? Having learned to answer these questions is what can make it possible for three-year-olds to understand and enjoy a 90+-minute feature film, probably with other family members, even if they then have to see it once or twice more to get all the meaning from it. And of course, it remains a set of skills that we continue to use throughout life as we not only view moving image media, but also read books, watch plays, and tell each other stories.

The slight liberalisation of "screen time rules," as represented by the AAP's shift of policy in 2016 and the EYSTAG advice ten years later may have involved some acknowledgment of the understandable difficulties that face any researchers who might want to establish reliable evidence about the longer-term effects of such a widespread and highly variable phenomenon as children's TV – and VOD-viewing. For research data to be convincing enough to justify universal rules such as the "screen time" requirements, they would have to be drawn from a very large sample of families. It is far too expensive and time-consuming for most research teams to visit hundreds of homes, even just to interview parents, let alone observe children's behaviour – and to interpret it correctly (not using assumptions based on prejudice, lack of knowledge of the child, or of the family's everyday behaviour) – and, even more complex and time-consuming, to follow up each child's development over many subsequent years. To prove that it is *just* the TV-watching that causes long-term effects, researchers would also have to gather evidence about family circumstances, such as income and employment. Another key factor that could relate to excessive "screen time" would be the nature and quality of relationships between family members (i.e. whether there's antagonism and stress), and that would be a lot harder to gather. Then researchers would have to spend several years closely following the later development, family circumstances, and school careers of children from a group of "heavy-viewing" families and compare them with another group of children from "light-viewing" families (having already carefully defined what they have decided to mean by "heavy" and "light," and assembled large enough groups of both types of family – at least several hundred of each) to provide some convincing proof that TV viewing *on its own* "can be" detrimental. Such a study would probably be interesting, and might be convincing, but it would also be unfeasibly complicated and expensive.

Some projects have managed to find reasonably large groups of parents by approaching families already involved in another project or in studies on health and development, but they would still have had to consider the complications I have just listed. More commonly, a large sample of families may be enrolled as volunteers for telephone interviews or written questionnaires. But few such researchers acknowledge the obvious unreliability of parental self-reporting as a starting-point for reaching trustworthy and generalisable conclusions. Any responses to questions such as "how much time does your baby spend in watching TV in a typical week?" are likely to be guesswork, unless the parents have been told in advance to note the amount of time spent, which then might easily result in the "timing week" being an untypical one anyway, because of the parents' heightened awareness of "screen time."

By the 2020s, public references to "screen time," and discussions about it, had almost completely refocused on teenagers and their social media use. In the UK, public awareness grew after the 2022 inquest on a teenager, Molly Russell, whose suicide was thought to be linked to the social media material she had been looking at. Three years later, the four-part Netflix series *Adolescence*, created by Jack Thorne and Stephen Graham, prompted another surge of public debate about teenagers' social media use, focused particularly on the notorious social media "influencer" Andrew Tate and how the concept of "incel" (involuntary male celibacy) could have negative effects on teenage boys. But after July 2025, an article by Zoe Kleinman on the BBC In Depth site (an arena for more extended investigations of news issues, and an invitation to respond) attracted nearly a thousand comments within two months. A central feature of Kleinman's article was her account of a book by a psychology professor at Bath Spa University, Pete Etchells, whose book *Unlocked: The Real Science of Screen Time,* is based on reviews of hundreds of studies on screen time and mental health, concluding that "concrete scientific evidence to back up stories about the terrible outcomes of screen time simply isn't there" and supports the fairly obvious case that social media provide benefits as well as risks to teens (Etchells, 2025).

But the issue of "screen time" for babies and toddlers continues to be debated from time to time on social media, especially by parents, not all of whom are persuaded by the kind of rules cited at the beginning of this chapter, and most of whom are probably unaware of the developing consensus amongst academics investigating teenagers' use of screens. Back in 2013, a paper by Duch, Fisher, Ensari, and Harrington had made comments, similar to Etchells' critique, about the effects of screens on teens. Here are their key findings:

- They had looked at 29 studies of "screen time," all but one of which relied on parents' *own* reports of how much "screen time" their children had in a "typical day": and they point out that self-reporting is very unlikely to be reliable. Few people are able to judge accurately the amount of time they usually spend on daily activities.
- They could not find, in *any* of the studies they reviewed, adequate information about key factors such as household income, parental education levels, mothers' ages – which could obviously affect the ways in which the children's activities were managed, as well as longer-term outcomes such as their health and educational achievement. In most of the studies, there was no information of this kind (Duch et al., 2013).

These were really important findings, and may also have contributed to the AAP's shift of policy in 2016. The report was also one of the 63 reviewed by the EYSTAG group that I discussed earlier in this chapter. It confirmed my own initial reactions to most of the pre-2013 debates and pronouncements on "screen time": that it doesn't make sense to isolate it as one factor in the child's upbringing, while ignoring much more significant factors that can have major negative effects on a child's emotional and intellectual development, such as parent/s being depressed and/or physically unwell, single parent families, poverty, the number and ages of children in the family, poor accommodation, and social isolation. Any of these factors – and, sadly, we know that some families might well have to endure two or more of them – are likely to mean that the parent/s affected by them would be more likely to depend on TV to occupy the child/ren while dealing with the other really challenging problems and worries that they had to face. These same factors would also be much more likely to have had a role in causing the alarming later "effects" in children's lives that many researchers have claimed to be the result of "excessive screen time," such as poor achievement in school, obesity, inability to concentrate, depression, and even problems in brain development.

While writing this book, I have twice been involved in social media threads on the topic of babies and toddlers' TV-watching: once on Mumsnet and once on my local Nextdoor.com group. I was not addressing the topic in general. In the Mumsnet thread, I simply asked "which is better: *Cocomelon* or *In the Night Garden*?" Within 24 hours there were 63 responses – the first one being "they're both rubbish" – but many of the others offered rhapsodic memories of watching *In the Night Garden* with their child/ren and a tendency to sneer at *Cocomelon*. In 2024, on my local Nextdoor.com, I contributed to an existing thread started by someone who was expressing shock and horror after having seen a baby looking at a mobile phone in a pram in some public place, to which I had responded with a brief attempt to suggest that this phenomenon might not be as terrible as many people think. I was rewarded with a shower of outrage and disgust, underlined with angry reminders that these warnings are "based on *scientific* evidence," implying that I must be stupid or naïve not to recognise the importance of science. Many knee-jerk-based debates about "science," such as the pro- or anti-vax arguments that followed the COVID pandemic in 2020, have indicated the understandable lack of public awareness about what actually does count as "trustworthy science," a confusion unfortunately fanned by a few high-profile figures such as Robert F. Kennedy Jr. Perhaps one of the major – and growing – issues of our time is that our schools must more adequately prepare people to make informed judgments about the claims for "scientific evidence" that we all constantly encounter.

TAKEWAYS

Double-checking

Do an online search, using the question "Is TV bad for babies?"

An online search for "Video Deficit Effect" will tell you how much progress has been made towards broader and more fully-informed accounts of the differences – and perhaps also the similarities! – between real-life encounters and relationships, and what we see on TV or VOD.

Further reading

Sonia Livingstone's useful account of changes in the "screen time" concept and the shift away from the AAP's "two hour" rule to an increase in advice about "good parenting" is available at https://blogs.lse.ac.uk/parenting4digitalfuture/2019/02/08/from-policing-screen-time/

Open letter to The Guardian by 80 academics: www.theguardian.com/science/head-quarters/2017/jan/06/screen-time-guidelines-need-to-be-built-on-evidence-not-hype

Etchells, P. (2025). *Unlocked: The real science of screen time*. Piatkus Books.

Woodhead, M., Faulkner, D., & Littleton, K. (1998). *Cultural worlds of early childhood*. New York: Routledge.

Observation

Try studying a child as s/he watches TV and consider what the challenges are in simply picking up small details of behaviour, and relating these to what s/he was watching at the time. As a parent, you might like to try videoing your child's viewing behaviour (you can do this quite unobtrusively with a phone – but DO create a wide frame by holding it "horizontally"!) and studying it yourself. It is inadvisable for Early Years practitioners to do this with other people's children, even with permission, for obvious ethical and legal reasons.

Discussion

If parents want to discuss a child's TV or VOD viewing with you, you need to be clear why, and to decide whether they would be receptive to the arguments made here. If they express anxiety or confusion about the advice they have been getting from friends, from their own parents, or from the media, you may feel it could be appropriate to refer to the arguments in this book. But be aware that this can be a fraught and complicated area to get into, unless you have an established relationship with the parent/s. Your safest strategy may be to follow the same advice as that now given by the UK's recent guidance, and by simply emphasising the "good parenting" advice that you are probably providing anyway. But look also at Chapter 9 for the value of viewing *with* child/ren when possible.

Strategies for HE contexts and training events

Ask students to recall their own childhood experiences of TV-watching and parental rules, if any. Asking about particular pleasures or fears can be a fruitful starting-point. Role-playing an argument between imagined couples can help students to envisage how they might manage strongly-felt attitudes.

References

Anderson, D. R., Alwitt, L. F., Pugzles Lorch, E. P., & Levin, S. R. (1979). Watching children watch television. In G. Hale & M. Lewis (Eds.), *Attention and cognitive development*. New York: Plenum Books.

Anderson, D. R., & Kirkorian, H. L. (2018). Effect of sequential video shot comprehensibility on attentional synchrony: A comparison of children and adults. *Proceedings of the National Academy of Sciences of the United States of America, 115*(40), 9867–9874. Retrieved from www.jstor.org/stable/26531356

Anderson, D. R., & Pempek, T. A. (2005). Television and very young children. *American Behavioral Scientist, 48*(5), 505.

Barber, S. E., Kelly, B. Collings, P. J., Nagy, L., Bywater, T., & Wright, J. (2017). Prevalence, trajectories, and determinants of television viewing time in an ethnically diverse sample of young children from the UK. *14*(88). Retrieved from https://ijbnpa.biomedcentral.com/articles/10.1186/s12966-017-0541-8)

Barr, R., Meuntener, P., & Garcia, A. (2007). Age-related changes in deferred imitation from television by 6- to 18-month-olds. *Developmental Science, 10*(6).

Calvert, S. L. (1988). Television production feature effects on children's comprehension of time. *Journal of Applied Developmental Psychology, 9*(3), 263–273.

Child Development Outcomes 2024-2025: Statistical commentary. (2025). London Department of Health and Social Care. Retrieved from www.gov.uk/government/statistics/child-development-outcomes-at-2-to-2-and-a-half-years-april-2023-to-march-2024-annual-2023-to-2024/child-development-outcomes-at-2-to-2-and-a-half-years-2023-to-2024-statistical-commentary

Duch, H., Fisher, E. M., Ensari, I., & Harrington, A. (2013). Screen time use in children under 3 years old: A systematic review of correlates. *The International Journal of Behavioral Nutrition and Physical Sctivity, 10*(1).

Etchells, P. (2025). *Unlocked: The real science of screen time (and how to spend it better)*: Piatkus.

EYSTAG. (2026). *Screen use by children aged under five: Independent report*. Retrieved from London.

Kirbas, S. I., & Smith, T. J. (2018). How infants perceive animated films. In M. Uhrig (Ed.), *Emotion in animated films*. London: Routledge.
Krcmar, M. (2010). Can social meaningfulness and repeat exposure help infants and toddlers overcome the video deficit? *Media Psychology, 13*(1), 31–53.
Lowe, P. J., & Durkin, K. (1999). The effect of flashback on children's understanding of television crime content. *Journal of Broadcasting and Electronic Media, 43*(1).
Nielsen, M., Simcock, G., & Jenkins, L. (2008). The effect of social engarement on 24-months-olds' imitation from live and televised models. *Developmental Science*, 11(5), 722–731. https://doi.org/10.1111/j.1467-7687.2008.00722.x
Simcock, G., Garrity, K., & Barr, R. (2011). The effect of narrative cues on infants' imitation from television and picture books. *Child Development, 82*(5), 1607–1619.
Sommer, K., Slaughter, V., Wiles, J., & Nielsen, M. (2023). Revisiting the video deficit in technology-saturated environments: Successful imitation from people, screens, and social robots. *Journal of Experimental Child Psychology, 232,* 105673. doi:https://doi.org/10.1016/j.jecp.2023.105673
Trevarthen, C. (1998). The child's need to learn a culture. In D. F. M. Woodhead, & K. Littleton (Eds.), *Cultural worlds of early childhood*. New York: Routledge.
Wass, S. V., & Smiht, T. J. (2015). Visual motherese? Signal to noise ratios in todder directed television. *Journal of Vision, 12*(1).

Chapter 3

The challenges of learning to understand moving image media

In 1992, the American scholar Edward Branigan asked an interesting question that has not been addressed by many other scholars:

> It seems remarkable that no one has undertaken to discover what special problems of narrative comprehension may be posed to a child by filmed narratives. For example, when and how do children understand an eyeline match, screen direction, cross-cutting, an unusual angle, off-screen space, or non-diegetic sound?
>
> (Branigan, 1992)

Perhaps his questions look unnecessarily technical, or even pretentious. The idea that moving image media are complicated systems that we have to learn to interpret may seem silly, given that most of us don't have any problems in understanding them. We enjoy the fact that films and TV can show us real places and real-looking fantasy ones, and behaviour that usually seems believable, even when it is weird or shocking.

Moving image media have come a long way from their first appearances in 1894/5. The earliest films were short, silent "documentary-style" black-and-white films that showed everyday events, without any cuts from one shot to another, and without any camera movement. Typical subjects were: a train arriving at a station, workers leaving a factory, the view from a bus moving along an ordinary street. We are told that audiences greeted them with cries of amazement or, in the case of the train moving towards them, screams of terror – though those claims may well have just been part the promotional efforts of early film-makers and exhibitors, rather than the documentary evidence they are usually claimed to be. Although the films were still clearly a form of photography (which had already existed for 75 years), the fact that they showed movement was an exciting development. But I wonder whether my grandfather's response might have been typical. He was 18 years old in 1895: in the 1960s, he told me that the early films were quite annoying to watch, being jerky and silent: quite *unlike* "real life." In this, his response

DOI: 10.4324/9781003751236-4

was similar to Maxim Gorky's 1896 review of the first films to be publicly exhibited: the Lumière Brothers' collection of short scenes:

> Their smiles are lifeless, even though their movements are full of living energy and are so swift as to be almost imperceptible. Their laughter is soundless although you see the muscles contracting in their grey faces. Before you a life is surging, a life deprived of words and shorn of the living spectrum of colours — the grey, the soundless, the bleak and dismal life.
>
> (Gorky, 1896)

Since then, there have been many technical and stylistic innovations in moving image media: camera movement, sound, colour, clearer definition, bigger screens – these have kept on drawing audiences closer into the action and making it all seem more "believable." People don't have to be regular TV viewers or cinema-goers to understand most of what they watch, and many of us now make our own videos on our phones, if only to convey a panorama of a holiday location or to share the playful activities of a child or a favourite pet. But few people have the knowledge and skills to edit their own videos. And it's annoying to see the amateur videos, made on phones, which get shown on TV when they are the only visual evidence of dramatic events, but are framed in "portrait" mode (i.e. by holding the phone "vertically") rather than "landscape" (holding it "horizontally") – thus omitting all the vital context!

It is the story-telling techniques that evolved in cinema during its first three decades that still form the basic "rules" of film language. They enabled film to break out of its early identity as just a lot of photographs that moved. Although there are now many different camera positions and various types of camera movement, as well as different ways of transitioning from shot to shot, you almost certainly know all of them already, even if you're not confident about naming them, and in any case most of the time you probably don't even notice them. But they are not difficult to identify, although they can be quite complicated to explain, which is why I've asked Barry Ecuyer to illustrate them. Most of them relate in some way to the ways in which we use and manage our own perceptions and their associated emotions in everyday life.

One of the many things that are ignored by the researchers I discussed in Chapter 2 is the fact that, like many art forms, the immediate appeal of moving image media is to the emotions. By that I don't mean at the simple level of the standard "big five" emotions: joy, sadness, fear, disgust, and anger (though of course films and TV can evoke those feelings) but the much more subtle responses that may be only fleetingly invoked, such as curiosity about what will happen next, revulsion towards an unpleasant character, or amusement at a funny one, shock at a dreadful news item. Emotional responses – some momentary, some overwhelming – are involved throughout all our engagements with cultural forms, and moving image media are no exception (Tan, 1996).

The rationale for the explanations of film techniques in this chapter is in support of my hypothesis that babies almost certainly don't understand them at first (up to three months, perhaps), and even when they can follow them, they may still be perplexed by the more complicated ones. I remember participating in a fascinating discussion with a group of teachers about whether a two-year-old might be able to interpret a "cut to close-up." One of them had asked "what if a two-year-old sees a shot of a ladybird on a leaf, which is then followed by a close-up of the ladybird? Does she think it's a different ladybird, or the same one but bigger?" We pondered this for quite a while, but agreed in the end that we didn't know, and couldn't figure out any way in which we might establish what the two-year-old might think. Kirbas and Smith's 2018 book chapter (Kirbas & Smith, 2018) provides an interesting discussion of this question, including a reference to a study of first-time viewers in Africa in the 1960s: they thought that the mosquitoes in close-up that they had been shown (as part of a campaign against malaria) were giant mosquitoes and so, since they didn't have any that looked like that, decided that they didn't need to protect themselves against the giant ones they'd been shown (Forsdale, 1966)

My opinion now is that a two-year-old with perhaps 18 months of TV-viewing behind her, would take the "cut to closeup" in her stride as part of the narrative she is following, but that a baby of, say, three months (the age at which my twin grandchildren started watching *In the Night Garden* and were, according to my daughter, "gobsmacked") will not understand it as part of a narrative, but will probably be finding it pleasurable enough, in the sense of intriguing, to go on viewing.

So in this chapter, I will describe how most of these techniques relate – some more closely than others – to the ways in which we manage our own perceptions, reflexes and emotions in everyday life. I argue that they must become familiar to children through repetition as they gradually learn to follow a narrative (see also Chapter 5) by re-watching short videos and by becoming familiar with one or more TV series. They thus learn them unconsciously, probably soon after they begin watching moving images which, as we know, is for most babies at some point in their first year. The only way of studying this learning process is to video child viewers' behaviour and study the results intensively, as I did with my grandchildren Connie and Alfie for my PhD research, although I began observing them properly when they were already 17 months old and had been watching TV regularly for well over a year. But because these techniques and devices do relate to our everyday real-life experiences and thought-patterns, we can assume that toddlers – and even babies – do get used to them by concentrating hard (as Sunu is doing in the photo at the beginning of Chapter 1) as well as through repeat viewings and extended commitments to single series.

Take the very simple and frequent device called "eyeline match." When a character in a film suddenly looks at something that is either out of the frame, or is somewhere in the scene but concealed from the audience (for example on the floor, or inside a drawer they've just opened) we expect that the next shot will show us what they are looking at. Sometimes this is a "cliff-hanger" shot at the end of an episode or a scene, and we have to wait for the next episode to find out what the next shot shows. However, baby-and-toddler TV and VOD don't have cliff-hangers. But the shot that follows the character's "sudden look" will almost certainly be what is called a "point-of-view shot" (or "POV shot"), because it shows us what the character has seen and reacted to, from their point of view. It may match what the story has led us to expect that the character will see, or it may be a complete surprise, to them and to us. Sometimes we don't get a POV shot after a character looks offscreen: we are just left to wonder what it is that they saw, until it is explained later in the narrative, or it might even be an end end-of-episode cliff-hanger. In Figures 3.1 and 3.2, Barry illustrates eyeline match with a pair of still images, but we hope you can see that it must be the skateboarder in Figure 3.2 that has distracted the boy in Figure 3.1.

The eyeline match is a very common device. It not only shows us what human interactions look like, but it also follows our own instinctive emotional behaviour. If I'm talking to someone and they suddenly break eye contact with me and look away in a different direction, my immediate instinct is to follow their gaze – often without consciously thinking about it – in order to find out what it is that they're looking at. We can imagine how important this has always been for humans – and for animals too, especially as a safety device or an indication of where there's food. When my cat is watching me, he notices when I turn my gaze to the "treats" packet. Thousands of years

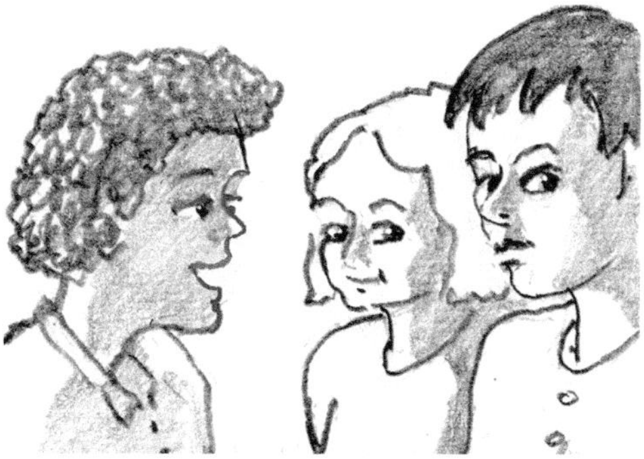

Figure 3.1 Eye direction 1.

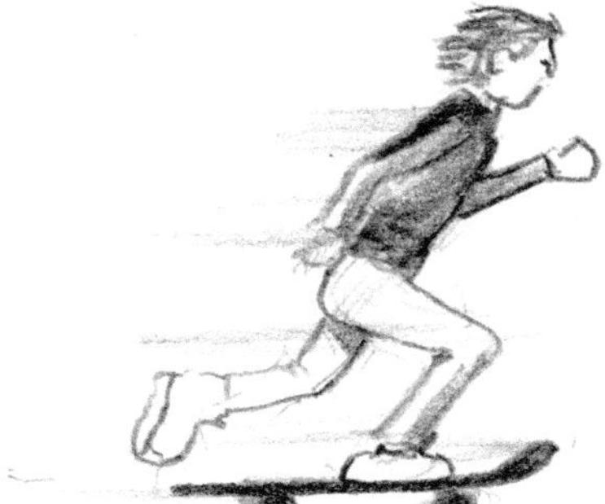

Figure 3.2 Eye direction 2.

ago, each member of a group of hunters or foragers would need to be constantly aware of what the others could see. And the use of a "cut" in the example I've just described expresses this more directly, even though it means that we instantly switch away from the original, "third-person" view of the character, to what we immediately understand to be a "first-person" point of view: what the character can see.

"Screen direction," the second item in Branigan's list, is also simple, but may seem complicated when explained. It refers to the need to maintain consistency, from one shot to another, with the directions in which characters or objects are moving. Let's say we see a person walking from *left to right* across the screen towards a closed door. We don't necessarily have to see them arrive at the door, grasp the handle, open the door and walk through, unless those movements are particularly significant at this point in the story (e.g. maybe we know – and the character doesn't – that opening the door will reveal something surprising or alarming). More often, there will just be a cut as the character approaches the door, and the next shot will show them coming through an open door into another room, or some other space. The important thing for maintaining narrative consistency, however, is that in the little sequence I've just described, the door that the character emerges through in the next shot must be on, or nearer to, the *left-hand side* of the screen, so that the character's movement maintains the same left-to-right direction in which they were walking in the previous shot. If the second shot showed the character emerging from a door on the right-hand side of the screen, we'd be confused: we'd get the impression that they'd suddenly turned around and started walking towards the left.

However, a film-maker might do that deliberately, as part of a specific narrative requirement. For example, the character walking towards the door in the first shot might be calling back to others in the room, saying something

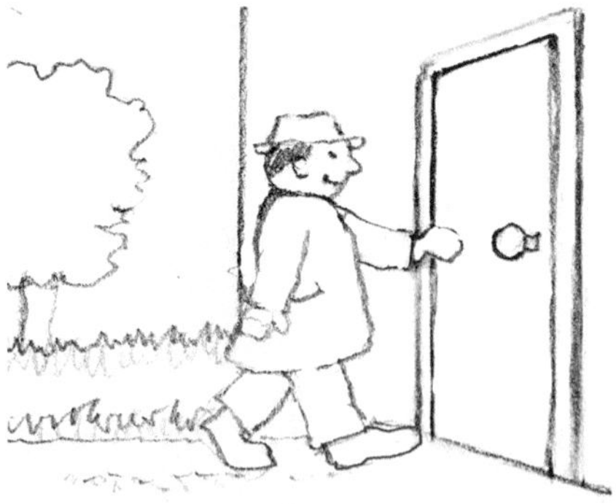

Figure 3.3 Screen direction 1.

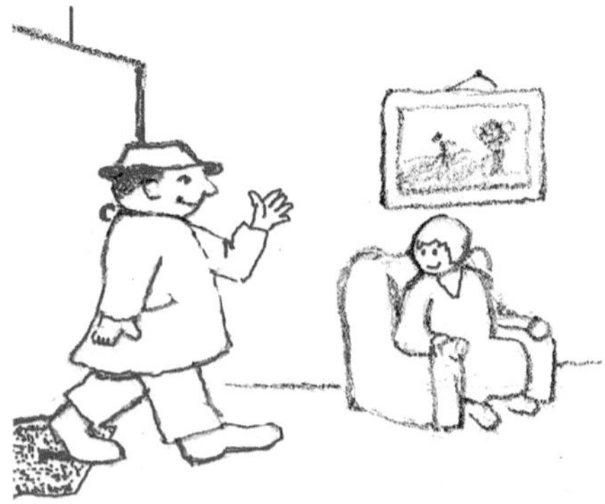

Figure 3.4 Screen direction 2.

like "I've gotta get over to Jim's place right away and tell him about this" If a following shot showed her coming through a door in a different position in the screen, it would be interpreted as happening later on, and somewhere else: viewers would realise that the character had arrived at Jim's place. That would be an example of another device: the "jump cut." This is when we can easily anticipate what is going to happen next in the story, so we don't need to be shown the boring bits in between, such as the character's journey to Jim's place.

Cross-cutting is sometimes called "parallel montage" or "parallel action." It involves switching between two action sequences that are happening at the same time: the classic example being shots of a woman tied to a railway track interspersed with shots of the approaching train and shots of the hero riding to save her (a suspense-inducing pattern which originally appeared in a weekly film serial called *The Hazards of Helen,* shown in cinemas in the USA between 1914 and 1917).

A cross-cutting build-up like this doesn't appear much, if at all, in baby or toddler channels and series, since the main point of the technique is to build up either agonising or comic suspense through repeated switching two and fro between two action sequences, which wouldn't be thought suitable for very young viewers, as well as being potentially confusing for them. The comic build-up in the puddle-splashing *Teletubbies* episode that I describe in Chapter 5 doesn't use cross-cutting: it's all filmed from one position. Cross-cutting isn't confined to action sequences: it could be used, for example, simply to compare the simultaneous activities of people in two different settings, which might be suspenseful, but could just be a way of comparing them or making a point: for example, shots of a person angrily tidying up a messy kitchen, cross-cut with shots of a teenager lying on a bed, idly scrolling through their phone.

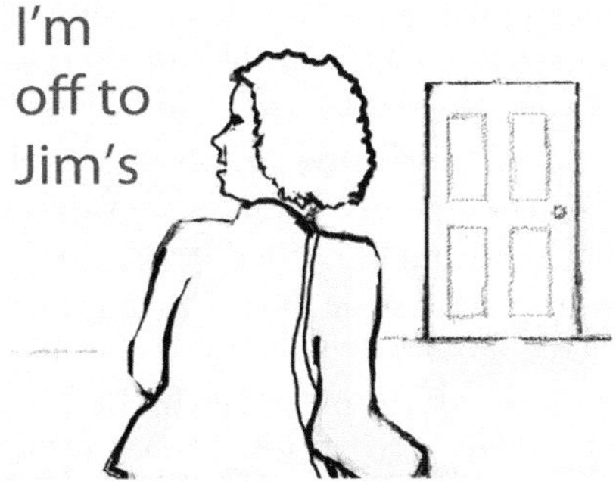

Figure 3.5 Screen direction 3.

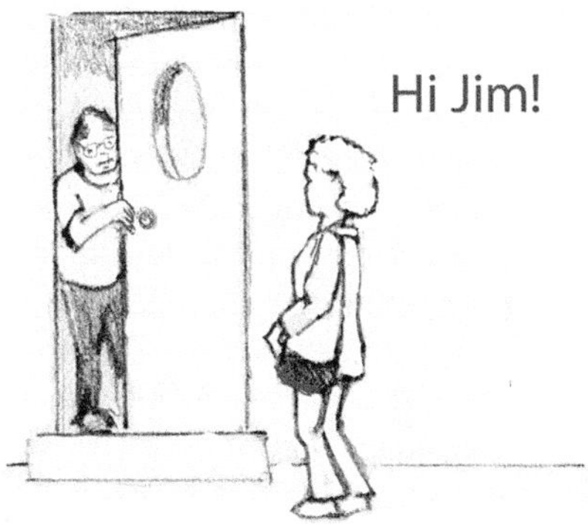

Figure 3.6 Screen direction 4.

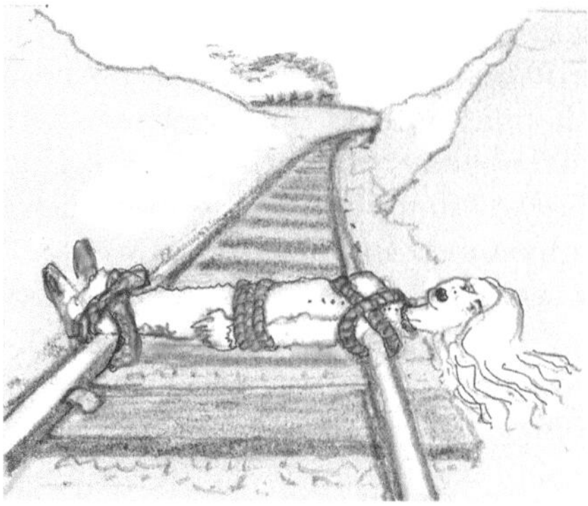

Figure 3.7 Cross-cutting 1.

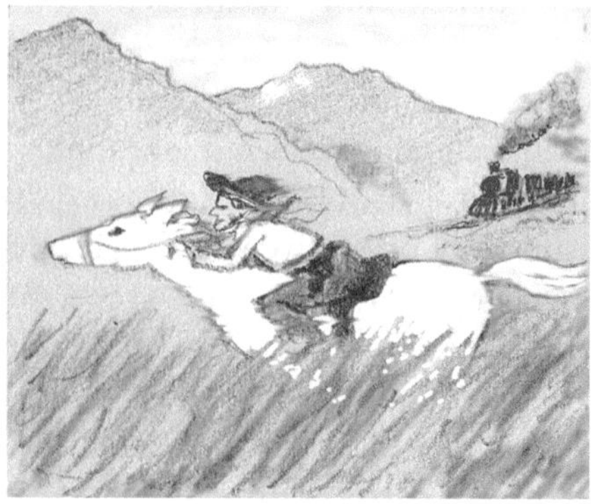

Figure 3.8 Cross-cutting 2.

Several different terms can be used to describe the "camera angle" or camera position: the way that a camera is set up to film a scene, or how an animator decides to frame a place or an actor. There are generally assumed to be around 8 camera positions that are commonly used, and are widely understood – such as "close up," "high angle," "medium shot," and so on. When Branigan refers to "an unusual angle" he presumably means rarer camera positions such as a tilted camera (or "Dutch angle" – which was used to indicate suspense or danger in some mid-20th century films, but is hardly ever used now). The choice of camera angle can often relate to the emotional tone of a scene: for example, a close-up of an excited face or tightly clenched hands. This isn't used much in TV for babies or toddlers, except perhaps as an indicator of surprise or pleasure. The shot of the oncoming train that would have followed the cross-cutting sequence that I described earlier would almost always be a "low-angle" shot, so more dramatic than the scene in Figure 3.9, which is more of a scene-setting image.

Off-screen space is an odd concept, since it only exists in the viewer's mind, but it is still important. If we are shown a particular space (a room, a boat, a space rocket) at the beginning of a sequence, but for the rest of the sequence the characters are shown sitting or standing close to each other and chatting, the viewer is likely to remain aware of the space that they are supposed to be in, and its location if that is established early on: this can be important to the story and to help us anticipate what will – or might – happen next, such as the door opening. This may sound complicated, but it is used a lot, even in baby TV programmes where there is an indoor setting, such as a living room, a nursery school classroom or a bus.

"Non-diegetic sound" might seem a very technical term, but it can be a useful one. The "diegesis" (pronounced "dyerJEEsis") of a film is the "world" it portrays: for example, the grassy, hilly landscape in the BBC TV children's series *Teletubbies* is an important part of the diegesis: it's the special place

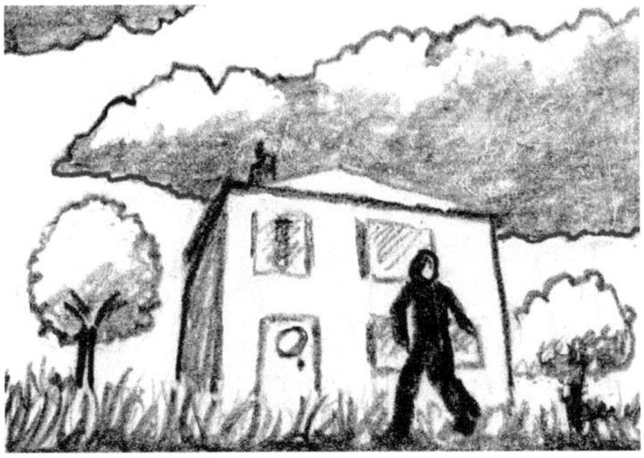

Figure 3.9 Low angle.

where much of the action happens. "Non-diegetic sound" is sound that you wouldn't expect to hear in the "world" of the film (i.e. it's a sound that we know the characters wouldn't be able to hear), but it does occur quite often in the form of thematic or background music. It can be heard in children's TV: for example, parts of *Peppa Pig* episodes are often accompanied by music that emphasises the light-hearted mood of the stories. Non-diegetic sound is satirised neatly and literally in Mel Brooks' 1974 film *Blazing Saddles*, where Sheriff Bart, riding across the desert with typical background music on the soundtrack, is amazed when he suddenly finds Count Basie's entire orchestra, sitting on chairs in the desert, actually playing it.

You may not want to bother remembering these terms, let alone use them, but I am confident that you already know what they refer to, even if you've never thought about them. I have explained them in rather laborious detail in order to emphasise how carefully and minutely all moving image stories are constructed – including programmes made for little children. I also want to emphasise children's achievement in the independent, self-driven learning that eventually enables them to understand what they watch on TV, phones. or tablets: for example, sequences of actions, character motivations. and reactions, the physical context of a scene. These devices may seem obvious to us, but they are not necessarily so for very young children. I remember seeing my son Ben, then aged about six months, sitting on my husband's lap as they both watched *Top of the Pops* (a weekly BBC programme, 1964–2006, showing performances of some of the week's best-selling popular music records). It often included shots that zoomed in on particular performers. I watched Ben moving his head steadily backwards as one performer's head started to fill the screen. Did it seem to him that the head was really getting bigger, or that he himself was somehow getting closer? No way of knowing – and no matter: this was simply a rare opportunity to actually witness a baby reacting (probably unconsciously) to a bit of "film language" that he presumably hadn't seen – or hadn't noticed – before, and it fascinated me at the time.

In "baby TV" programmes, this device and at least some of the others mentioned by Branigan (which I'll come back to in later chapters) are likely to be repeated often, thus helping babies to learn how to understand the language of moving images. *Cocomelon*'s 18-minute animated version of "The wheels on the bus go round and round" makes up for what some of us may have come to consider a tediously repetitive and over-familiar song, by using all of the devices that Branigan mentions: eyeline match, screen direction, cross-cutting, unusual angles, off-screen space, and the non-diegetic sound of the music. They serve to establish what the driver is doing (turning the wheel, opening and shutting the doors, beeping the horn, etc); and where the passengers are sitting in relation to each other: the family (mum, dad and three children) and the five animals (bear, pig, monkey, cat. and elephant) who get on the bus at the next stop.

I think it is likely – but maybe impossible to establish through research – that some devices are much easier than others for a baby to understand. For example, travelling shots, which replicate a character's point of view as they move through a scene (e.g. through a crowd, along a road, moving from one room to another in a building, etc.) may well be easy for babies to understand, given that they are constantly being carried or pushed in a buggy and are used to watching the world go by, and to seeing objects, scenery or people coming towards them before passing out of their field of vision. A series of cuts from one character to another may take a bit longer to figure out, as may cuts between long-shots and close-ups, and cuts from one scene to another. In my Chapter 10 analyses of *Cocomelon* and *Bluey*, I refer to some of these devices in context.

Maybe you are thinking that all this stuff about film language is a bit nerdy – unnecessary, in other words: as in "why don't they just shut up and enjoy the film?" I have a counter-argument to this, taken from one of our experiences in the British Film Institute's Education Department. In the early 2000s we were working with local authority education advisers and schools across England, to encourage teaching about film in primary schools. The project involved providing training courses for the teachers who were keen to learn how to teach about film. We created, and gave them, DVDs of carefully researched and selected short films, mostly from independent film-makers, that we were confident would appeal to primary age children, and taught them techniques for analysing and discussing them with their classes. Many of the teachers were dubious at first about whether their students would enjoy the films because they were almost certainly very different from what they usually saw, and even more dubious about whether they could be persuaded to watch them more than once and discuss them in class.

But when these teachers reported back on their first sessions in their classrooms they were always, without exception, flabbergasted by how enthusiastic all the children had been, and even more amazed by the transformations they had seen, not only in the children's willingness but also in their previously unsuspected abilities: to talk eagerly, comment perceptively, analyse the films they had seen and view them more than once. Very often, they had subsequently begun to write stories far more creatively than they had usually done. "They used words we didn't know they knew!" exclaimed one teacher (referring to new vocabulary that the children started using in their own writing; we didn't ask them to teach technical terms about film-making). But the children had been excited to hear that things they'd often noticed in films were important, well-known techniques, with special names. Some of them even adapted techniques in their writing that were similar to film language: vividly describing a character's point of view, for example. Most of them probably had, after all, been viewing TV programmes and films since they were toddlers or even younger, but had never been encouraged to think about how they were made, and had never seen films that were stylistically unusual.

To return to Branigan's question, is it possible to answer "when and how" children come to understand the devices that film-makers use in their stories? I think the short answer is that it is probably impossible to pinpoint the "when" bit, at least in a way that could be predicted at a particular developmental stage and apply to all children, since they don't all watch the same things. But it is possible to offer a simple answer to the "how" bit: they learn through watching things repeatedly and probably by thinking about them, or remembering them, as well. And in some cases, it may be that a parent or carer has commented on what they were watching or talked them through a scene they hadn't understood. I come back to this in Chapter 4, because some parents worry about what appears to be "obsessive" or "addictive" behaviour, and therefore I think it's probably worth encouraging consideration of what "learning film language" must involve and what it may look like in the child's behaviour.

But it is also more than this. Films aren't just constructed to show us things or to provide information. They are cultural artefacts and therefore they also work on our emotions. I referred earlier to Tan's 1996 book, *Emotion and the Structure of Narrative Film*, in which he refers to films as "emotion machines" (Tan, 1996), stating that "we cannot understand how a viewer grasps a cut between two shots, let alone a longer sequence of shots, without assuming that some mental structure is in operation, one that has been made active by the narration" (p X). Although he confines his study to feature films between 1920 and 1960, what he has to say is just as relevant to baby TV and how it is watched. Films – including animated films – contain characters, towards whom viewers quickly develop feelings. These may be merely recognition of what their role is – "this one looks like he might be the bad guy" – or we may find them immediately attractive, not just physically but as likeable, sympathetic characters. They also show scenes that will seem familiar to many child viewers, such as the argument between Bluey's parents that I describe in Chapter 10.

In baby TV, the bonds between characters and viewers are extremely strong right from the outset, because characters often appear to be looking at the viewer, with their big eyes, replicating – on an exaggerated scale – the wide-eyed, direct gaze that most of us immediately and instinctively offer to a baby we meet for the first time, saying something like "Hallo! Aren't you gorgeous!" and are delighted when they respond by meeting our gaze and perhaps even smiling. And of course, eye contact, and the various emotional responses it generates, is vitally important in almost all of our interpersonal experience. We pick up emotional cues, even from momentary encounters in the street, which can be intriguing: friendly, unfriendly, anxious, preoccupied, sad, fearful. It follows therefore that when a character in a baby TV show looks offscreen, baby viewers aged three months or more may start expecting the next shot to be what the character is looking at. Babies and toddlers won't at first notice the more complex ones such as screen direction or non-diegetic sound, and these are rarely used in baby TV anyway. But as they start to become more familiar with TV conventions – and, of course, by doing a lot of repeat-viewing and sticking for some time to one preferred series – their emotional responses to what they watch will develop, just as their social awareness of the people around them is also developing. They will care about some characters, share in their emotional states: being anxious about their anxieties, for example, and delighted when they solve a problem. This is after all the major function of cultural forms: as adults, we may seek out novels, plays, paintings, poems, films, and TV series that promise to affect us emotionally, including those that make us weep.

I was shocked when I started my PhD research and looked at the first video I made (which you can see on Vimeo at https://vimeo.com/bazalgette). It was quite a surprise for me at the time. It shows my granddaughter Connie, aged 21 months, starting to watch a programme called "Mr Bloom's Nursery" (BBC CBeebies 2011–2013) which is a rather excitable, full-on entertainment featuring a lot of characters including live action with "Mr Bloom" (played by Ben Faulks), real children, music, songs, and animated vegetables. Soon after the programme began, in contrast to the busy action on screen, Connie slid off the sofa, walked up to the coffee table that was positioned in front of the TV, rested one hand on the table, and a maintained a serious expression on her face, watching the screen intently (see Figure 3.10).

She stayed standing and absolutely motionless for the remaining four minutes of the programme, and then continued to watch a series of shots of children in playgrounds, and the jolly CBeebies presenters, only finally relaxing and moving away from the table after she'd been watching, almost motionless, for over seven minutes. She had ignored her grandfather's suggestion that she dance to the music, and her twin brother Alfie's more casual and

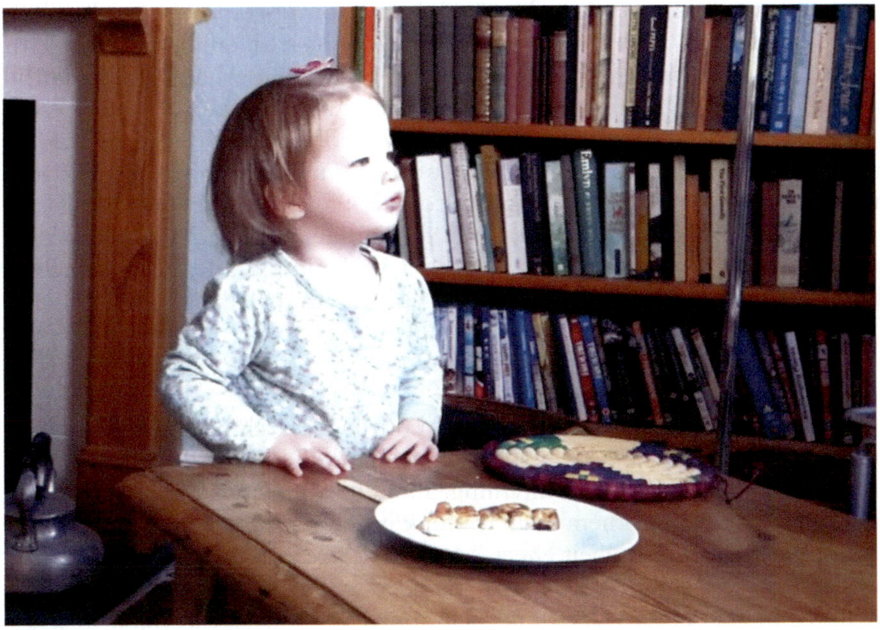

Figure 3.10 Connie watching TV.

intermittent viewing behaviour. I hadn't anticipated that my research might involve studying the tiny details of a child's intently focused viewing, rather than the livelier interactions I'd been expecting, and that Alfie did present on that occasion, although in most subsequent viewing he also concentrated and stayed still. This presented me with quite a challenge: I realised that I'd need to make video the centre of my observational work, and to study these videos extremely closely, in the way that I've demonstrated with Figure 1.1 in Chapter 1. And I would need to think about why the children often seemed to be concentrating so hard as they watched.

A baby's or toddler's early viewing experiences are certain to include at least some of the devices I've described earlier in this chapter. So we need to try and imagine what it feels like to encounter, for the first time, a device such as a point-of-view shot. For example, we might see a close-up of a child's face, whose eyes and mouth are both opening wide, not looking at the camera but in another direction. We then get a wider shot of a plate of delicious-looking cakes on a table. It's obvious to me or you that the child was reacting to the sight of the cakes. But is it obvious to a baby? Might he want to see it again to figure out what's going on? But he's then confronted by other shots: perhaps a wide-shot view of the room where the table is, this time showing several other children jumping up and down in excitement. Meanwhile the sound-track may include the sounds of voices, perhaps as well as music – instrumental, or a song, or both. And almost immediately there will be more: perhaps a differently-angled shot of an adult encouraging the children to choose a cake each, or even a completely different wide-angle shot of everyone reaching for a cake. For us this would all look quite ordinary and obvious, but to a first-time viewer it could seem quite complex and would reward a second or even third viewing, to work out the momentum and motivations at work in what we adults might see as a very simple and familiar scene. The *Cocomelon* "wheels on the bus" episode that I referred to earlier is far more complicated and fast-moving, with many different angles, and at one point, a bit of a story involving one of the children. It is likely to reward frequent re-viewings.

One of the problems with a great deal of the research on children and TV or "screen time," is that, as I explained in Chapter 2, many of the researchers not only don't know much, if anything, about how moving image media make meanings, but most of them seem to think it doesn't matter. In the Chapter 2 section on the "video deficit effect," I described researchers' attempts to differentiate between children's ability to understand some instructions given to them by a person in a video, and their ability to understand similar instructions given by someone with them in the same room. They didn't use existing online or broadcast material for the video, but presumably had the video made in their own research facility, perhaps hiring an actor. Inevitably, these made-to-order videos were nowhere near the standard of professionally-made material. They still might have intrigued children for a while simply because they would have been so different from what they were used to, but it is equally likely that they would have seemed a bit dull compared to the more exciting things the children had probably seen on TV. Either way, it seemed that the children didn't understand the video instructions, and this was taken to mean that children cannot learn from video: hence the concept of the "video deficit effect" which is sometimes still quoted as a "scientific fact" – for example it is referred to in several of the links I received in an online search about the question "is TV bad for babies?" (see Chapter 2). The possibility that none of us will learn much from something that is boring and/or peculiar didn't come up. The bizarre implication of this experiment is that the researchers seemed to have assumed that "video" is all the same. The fact that it was moving images was for them the important thing, the possibility of having different shots and using different ways of motivating and linking them, was not seen as important.

This is why another "danger" that is frequently cited by researchers and by the organisations that warn of TV's allegedly "bad effects" is that children don't learn anything useful or important *from* their TV-viewing. They are referring exclusively to numbers and words: television, they say, does not help children to become articulate and numerate. Apart from the fact that there are several TV programmes and series that are intended to do exactly that (especially in public-service provision), this alleged "danger" completely ignores the kind of learning that I have described in this chapter: how to understand a medium that is an important part of modern culture, reflects so many aspects of human behaviour and interaction, and can affect our emotions in many ways. It fails to appreciate the extraordinary self-driven learning that babies and toddlers undertake as soon as they start to try and make sense of what has become a rich and complex medium.

A rather more paranoid argument is made on the widely quoted American website www.raisewildflowers.com. This is run by Jessica Sannes, an American mother, who displays remarkable levels of hostility to baby/toddler TV shows. They are, she warns "so overstimulating that they actually act as a drug, a stimulant," and that any children who watch them "experience very real symptoms of addiction and withdrawal, which understandably leaves them emotionally dysregulated" – ignoring the possibility that anyone would get annoyed if someone else suddenly turned off a programme they were watching, or snatched away an interesting book. Sannes even claims that "the more a child is exposed to these types of shows, the more their brain begins to crave and expect this intense level of stimulation, making it impossible for them to play creatively and without entertainment." Her main basis for this seems to be that her own son became contrary and "difficult" when he started watching TV, though one wonders whether this was merely the start of his "terrible twos" phase (more about the alleged contrariness of this phase in the next chapter): if so, it could be that he needed to watch something repeatedly in order to make better sense of it, but she stopped him doing so, and he was understandably furious.

Almost certainly, most of us have experienced the process of becoming temporarily enthusiastic about a particular genre of films, or novels, or indeed any cultural product, such as a particular type of shoe, recipe, décor – the list is endless! And Sannes' claim that these shows are "carefully designed to hold a young child's attention" makes one wonder whether she has ever read a book, watched a film, or been to the theatre. It would be hard to find any form of storytelling or entertainment that has not been carefully designed to hold one's attention, and we all hope that we can hold people's attention effectively, whether we are speaking to an audience, telling a funny story to a friend, or writing a book. The problem with Sannes' type of cod psychology is that it doesn't recognise the huge and significant role of *culture* in the lives of all humans – including babies and toddlers. My aim in this chapter has simply been to demonstrate that film and TV are indeed carefully designed to hold our attention. In fact, I did carefully design this chapter to try and hold your attention. If you've got this far, it must have worked!

TAKEAWAYS

Brief experiments

a Try monitoring your own posture and bodily tension for five minutes while you try to keep perfectly still as you watch something engrossing on TV, or scroll through some important messages on your phone, or listen to a thrilling piece of music. Do you need to make any movements before the five minutes are up?

b Review any temporary enthusiasms you've had in your life: for example, a fashion fad you had when you were 16? A temporary devotion to a musical genre or a specific group? A book you loved and re-read? Can you remember what attracted you to them at the time? Or why you moved on to something else?

c If you are caring for one or more children, in a context where TV-viewing is possible, practicable, and approved by parents and/or carers, try observing them as they watch and noting what they are doing. It could be particularly interesting to observe them watching a short film or a series episode for the first time.

d You – and children, might be very briefly amused to watch Edison's 1894 film *Kinetoscopic Record of a Sneeze* (www.youtube.com/watch?v=2wnOpDWSbyw) but don't blink, as it lasts barely five seconds (and there's no sound track)!

e *Film language*

  i If these five techniques are new to you and you feel uncertain about what they are, and/or you want to understand them better, visit a website such as https://industrialscripts.com/cinematic-language/ to watch examples of these and others, with commentary.

  ii Try noting the techniques in use while you are watching a streamed TV drama (so that you can stop, rewind and re-view if you are uncertain about whether you have identified them correctly) and think about how they work. In each case, could there have been more than one way of conveying the meaning?

Further reading

Branigan, E. (1992). *Narrative comprehension and film*. Routledge.

Lancaster, L. (2001). Staring at the page: The functions of gaze in a young child's interpretation of symbolic forms. *Journal of Early Childhood Literacy*, *1*(2), 131–152 is about still images but is a fascinating and sympathetic account of a child's intense attention.

Monaco, J. (1977; 2009). *How to read a film*. Oxford University Press.

References

Branigan, E. (1992). *Narrative comprehension and film*. New York: Routledge.
Forsdale, F. (1966). Film literacy. *Journal of the University Film Producers Association, 18*(3).
Gorky, M. (1896). The kingdom of shadows. Retrieved from www.mcsweeneys.net/articles/contest-winner-36-black-and-white-and-in-color
Kirbas, S. I., & Smith, T. J. (2018). How infants perceive animated films. In M. Uhrig (Ed.), *Emotion in animated films*. London: Routledge.
Tan, E. S. (1996). *Emotion and the structure of narrative film: Film as an emotion machine*. Mahwah, NJ: Lawrence Erlbaum Associates.

Chapter 4

Not "terrible twos" but "dedicated learners"

When an Italian friend pointed out to me one day that there's no equivalent of the term "terrible twos" in Italian, I started wondering about how attitudes to children may vary from one culture to another, and whether the words or expressions that may be used in different languages to describe two-year-olds might be a "way in" to finding that out. So far, I've asked native speakers of 15 languages other than English: all were certain that their language did not contain a term anything like "terrible twos.." A German did admit that they call the third year of life "the age of defiance," and an academic colleague from Spain had found that some languages are starting to adapt "terrible twos" because of its widespread use in English. So, are English two-year-olds especially terrible? Or is it English-speakers (including Americans) who are more likely to perceive two-year-olds as terrible? If so, why? And in any case, what is the nature of the "terribleness" to which at least some people refer?

Like other parents and grandparents, I've become used to the fact that, as toddlers become more mobile, dextrous, and talkative, they have a lot more resources for insisting on their own preferences and demands. So what the "terrible twos" label refers to is usually violent expressions of frustration or resistance, especially when they are asked (or ordered, or forced) to stop doing something. This can be when they are, or may be about to be, doing something dangerous. But more often, it is because we want them to stop doing one thing and start doing something else that we think is more important: get ready to go out, get back in the buggy, put that toy away, etc. To understand the reasons for toddlers' desperate insistence on what they want to do, we have to go back a long way: maybe even to pre-humans. More detail on most of what follows can easily be found online, in Wikipedia, and many other sites.

There is some discussion amongst anthropologists and other experts on human development and anatomy, about a hypothesis called "the obstetrical dilemma." The problems that it addresses do exist, even if the causes of them remain debatable. The starting-point is claimed to be the established fact that, as humans gradually evolved from apes over a six-million-year period,

DOI: 10.4324/9781003751236-5

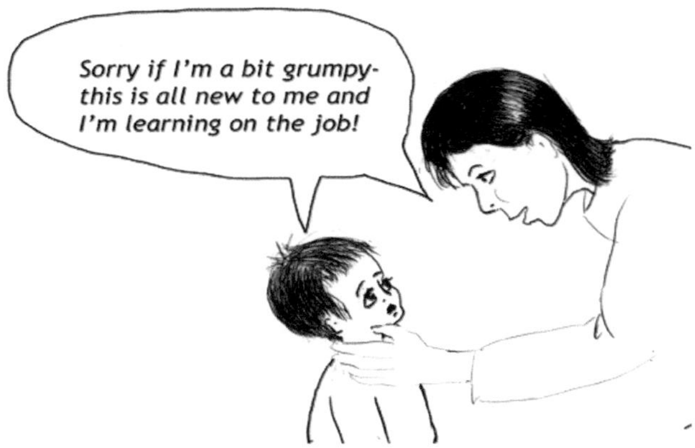
Sorry if I'm a bit grumpy-
this is all new to me and
I'm learning on the job!

Figure 4.1 Terrible Twos?

one of the key developments in that process – which in itself took around two million years – was the gradual development of a primate species that naturally and habitually walked and ran on two legs rather than four. Although these Australopithecines could not have continued to climb trees as easily as apes can, or run as fast, their front feet had developed into hands with opposing thumbs, that could manipulate small or complicated objects. That enabled them to make more elaborate tools than the "nut-cracking" and "stick-poking" types of tools that apes can make and use. They therefore gained advantages over apes, so their populations started to grow, and over the next million years or so, their abilities to see further, and to think, discover, and plan ahead, continued to develop.

Over the same period, however, the pelvic bones and skulls of these bipedal, dextrous creatures also gradually changed shape, and this is where the "obstetric dilemma" discussion comes in. Some specialists argue that walking and running on two legs doesn't work that well if you have a very wide pelvis, as chimpanzees, gorillas, and other apes still do. So according to that argument, the Australopithecines soon became more successful than those with wider hips. Walking on two legs freed up their front feet to develop into hands, which meant that, over time, they gained the abilities needed to make weapons and tools for killing and butchering prey as well as developing wider shoulders. Whether or not this is an accurate account of their development, it's certainly true that all humans today do have relatively narrow hips and wider shoulders (Laudicina & Cartmill, 2023), compared to the great apes. Over the same long period, the dextrous hominins began to make tools, solve problems, and communicate with one another through eye-contact and gestures and, later, spoken language. Consequently, over the next two million or more years it was the ones whose brains (and therefore their skulls) became bigger, whose populations really began to grow as they continued to evolve and began to spread away from Africa to other parts of the world, becoming what we now acknowledge as human.

So "being human" may have come at a price: the combination of narrow pelvises, wide shoulders, and big heads means that human childbirth is more dangerous for human mothers and babies than it is for any other mammal. We are what is called an "altricial species": the only human babies who can survive childbirth are those that are still small enough to pass through the mother's narrow pelvis, as long as they turn sideways during birth so that their shoulders can also pass through. But that means they are helpless as well as small: in fact, they're premature! And of course, that then means they need continuous care and attention. Human babies can't get up and walk soon after birth, like new-born calves or lambs, and although their fingers do instinctively grasp, they can't support their own weight by holding on to their mother's hair while she runs or climbs, as baby chimpanzees, bonobos, and orang-utans can. Nevertheless, it's not necessary to regard this as a problem. We humans have still managed to survive in large enough numbers to populate most of the planet's land-masses and, indeed, to threaten its future by exploiting its resources too extravagantly. But alongside our development of bipedalism, tool use, cooperation, and language, we must always have been tender and ingenious carers of our feeble little offspring, and our babies must have always been fast learners, or the inexorable processes of evolution would have finished us off thousands of years ago.

Human babies are born with a few instincts: to turn their heads and suckle, to grasp, to recognise their carer(s). They need a huge amount of care, but nevertheless they immediately start to learn. They are soon able to roll over, manipulate objects (starting with their own hands!), and to recognise sounds and surroundings. New surfaces and textures must be felt and explored, new people assessed, new contexts understood, new sounds imitated. What babies can also do, from the start, is to socialise. Experts tell us that new-borns can't focus or see very far, but it did seem absolutely certain to me (and other mothers have told me of similar experiences) that my new-born son and I did, very briefly, gaze intently at each other when he was less than ten minutes old, in the arms of a midwife standing beside the bed (the birth had been difficult: I was still lying down and hadn't been given him to hold). One thing that new-borns definitely do already know is the sound of their mother's voice. They have been hearing it, as well as sounds from outside her body, from the third month of the pregnancy. So for babies, birth must also include the revelation of suddenly seeing the creatures who'd been making these sounds: people! Now they can start trying to integrate their aural experiences with their new senses of sight and touch, and, before long, to begin making sense of the culture they have been born into: starting perhaps, at around six weeks, with their first real, social smile: at someone who is smiling at them.

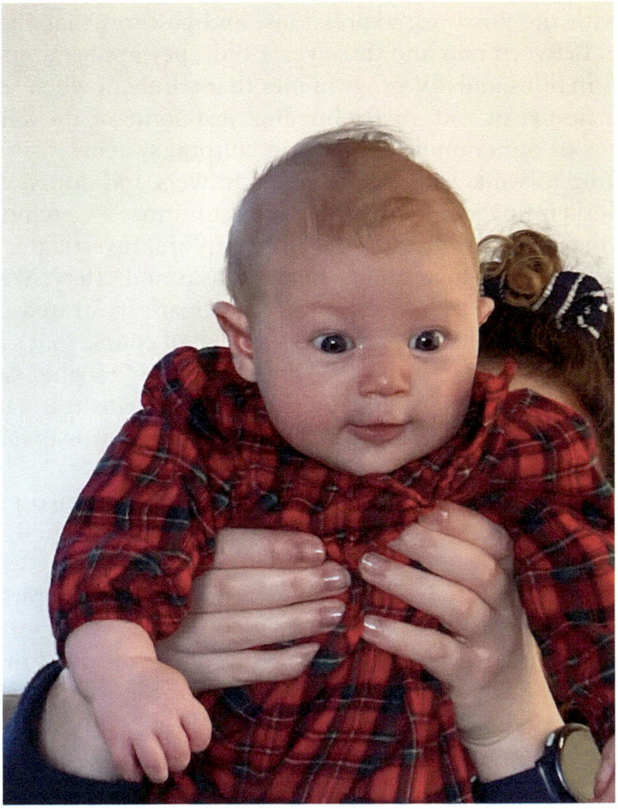

Figure 4.2 Evie at seven weeks. Photo: Caroline Mitchell.

Over their first few weeks, babies' curiosity about the people and things they see around them becomes ever more intense. By six weeks old, they have learned to smile, responding to the smiles of others; years later, most of us probably smile instinctively when we briefly lock eyes with a stranger making way for us in a crowded bus or train, or make eye contact with a baby or toddler in a buggy. The seven-week-old baby in Figure 4.2 has become practised at turning her head, focusing on objects and people, expressing fascination and delight.

It is these gazes and intense responses that bond us to our children from birth onwards. We are an intensely social species – which also means that we have developed artefacts, languages, and cultural traditions. During their second year of life, toddlers learn enough of a language – or maybe two languages if they're available: it's not hard to learn that everything has two names! – to communicate what they want and don't want, to ask questions, and to identify things and people. Mimes, clowns, and silent films can entertain toddlers with the postures, expressions, and gestures that they've learned to recognise. Between two and three years old, they are beginning to understand the clues in films and TV programmes that tell them when something is going to be funny, or sad, or frightening: just some of the simple, easy-to-learn elements of our complicated human cultural systems.

Toddlers are starting to walk and talk, to open drawers and doors, carry objects around, stick their fingers into apertures and substances. Catching up on that early birth, they have an incessant need to explore, investigate, test, and discover, which far exceeds their ability to judge risks and safety. We can better tolerate their rage when these exploratory urges are frustrated if we can keep in mind the intensity of their curiosity – though of course that's hard to do when they're poised on the brink of danger. But the "terrible twos" concept pushes the idea that their behaviour is wilful and selfish. It can let tired parents feel that their child is doing it on purpose: that they just want to be perverse and annoying.

If the "terrible twos" concept really is almost completely confined to the speakers of English, as my informal investigations have so far indicated, why it this? Could it be related to Britain's history? By the 19th century, Britons boasted that their colonising activities had created "the biggest empire the world has ever seen." I remember as a child in the 1940s leafing excitedly through an atlas to see how many parts of the world were coloured in red, and were therefore "ours." Many historians have pointed out that, from the 16th century, British colonisers felt justified in seizing the territories of what they saw as "primitive" or "backward" peoples, because, as the 17th-century Puritan leader John Winthrop observed of Indigenous people in the Americas, "they inclose no land, neither have they cattle to maintain it, but remove their dwellings as they have occasion" (Lepore, 1998); so the colonialists saw the lands they had invaded as "vacant," to be exploited any way they wished. In 1870, John Ruskin gave his inaugural lecture in Oxford about England's "duty" to colonise the world, in which he similarly characterised Indigenous land as "waste." His often-quoted message to "England" was:

> This is what she must either do, or perish: she must found colonies as fast and as far as she is able, formed of her most energetic and worthiest men; seizing every piece of fruitful waste ground she can set her foot on, and there teaching these her colonists that their chief virtue is to be fidelity to their country, and that their first aim is to be to advance the power of England by land and sea.
>
> (full text at https://en.wikisource.org/wiki/Inaugural_Lecture)

In his book *Empireland*, Sathnam Sanghera describes how closely linked the English public school system was to the administration of the British Empire (Sanghera, 2021). It became a prime function of these schools in the 19th and early 20th centuries to turn out the sort of young men, many of whom were going to be colonists, who would be able to administer the colonies efficiently, and deal confidently with the black and brown people whom they were encouraged to see as undisciplined, ignorant "natives," often characterised – sometimes affectionately, but usually condescendingly or dismissively – as "childlike," at least when they weren't being regarded as "primitive," and could be sentimentally admired, or brutally massacred. Victorian attitudes to children were therefore close to the ways in which the British imagined and defined Indigenous people. Perhaps it is not a coincidence that the motto "children should be seen and not heard," while not unique to English, is particularly associated with Victorian Britain. Even now it's often acceptable, in middle-class British culture, to raise the objection "but it'll be full of screaming kids" in conversations about choosing a restaurant, park, or holiday destination; and common for those who oppose that argument to point out how surprisingly welcome little children are in French, Spanish, Italian, or Greek restaurants and cafés (even though they had also been imperialist cultures).

The basis of my argument in this book is that almost everything toddlers do (when they're awake, at least!) is motivated by their urge to learn. We obviously try to ensure that they don't learn some things the hard way (hot water can scald your fingers, floor polish tastes horrible, knives can cut you, etc.), but when they are clearly fascinated by something and determined to figure out what it is, it can be fascinating to us as well – when we can – to let that process take its course. My reaction to something that my other grandson, Morgan, was doing when he was about two and a half is an example of this. One evening I noticed him "playing" (as I assumed) with a double-socket power point that had three plugs in it, two attached to an adapter. It wasn't at floor level but on the wall close to a chair, so Morgan must have had to climb up in order to stand there and investigate it. As I approached to tell him not to play with it, "it's not a toy" etc., I suddenly realised that he was very carefully turning the switches on and off, because they were connected to the three lamps that stood in different places around the room. One switch turned two lights on and off; the other only operated one. He had to look closely at the switches to turn them on and off, and each time he had to turn and look round the room to see which one affected which light(s). He was experimenting: he had to try both switches, several times, until he had found out which one did what. So I hovered: nervously, but increasingly fascinated. He was, of course, outraged when I made him stop and have his dinner.

When one has the time, it is worth trying to observe and reflect on what a child is doing when she is examining something very closely. For example, I was intrigued by the implications of the behaviour shown in Figure 4.3, and the drawing shown in 4.4. Both relate to children's concept of scale, but in contrasting ways. Figure 4.3 displays what I think is quite common behaviour: it shows Alfie, aged 26 months, lying down beside a toy train on its track, trying to visualise it as a full-size train. It shows his consciousness of

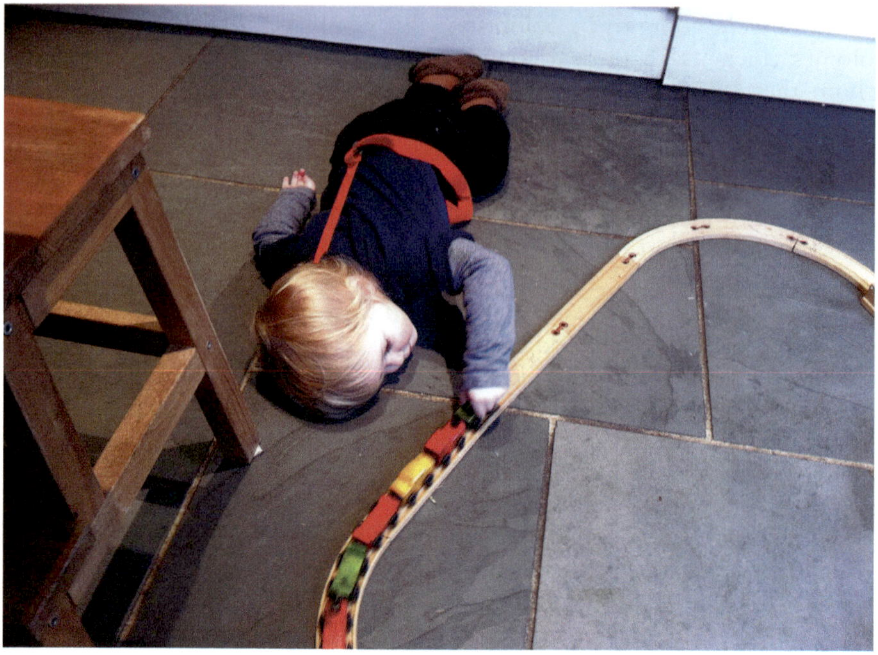

Figure 4.3 Scale: Alfie makes the train look bigger. Photo: Cary Bazalgette.

scale and his efforts to imagine what the toy represents. In contrast, Figure 4.4 is a typical three-year-old's representation of his family, showing his parents and himself as all the same size, all consisting only of immensely long legs, with small heads on top. This style of figure-drawing may seem grotesque to us, but is of course how we appear to toddlers: very tall, with heads that are far away! The dots on the image are from the many times it was proudly pinned up to be admired. I did wonder, when I realised that both these images involve boys, whether male toddlers are more interested in relative sizes than girls are. There is a huge amount of research literature on children's play and toys, and on gender differences in their behaviour: Davis and Hines have a very extensive bibliography for their interesting article (Davis & Hines, 2020), but although there are some striking gender-related toy preferences, I didn't find anything about gender-related preoccupations with scale.

Most children seeing a TV programme or video for the first time are immediately curious, as they are with anything new, but – as I argued about four-month-old Sunu's posture and expression in the picture at the beginning of Chapter 1 – intense concentration indicates a stronger commitment than just curiosity, even in a four-month-old – and that was not her first encounter with *Cocomelon*. When they view TV or VOD, the size of the figures and the differences in sizes between adult and child figures must be important and

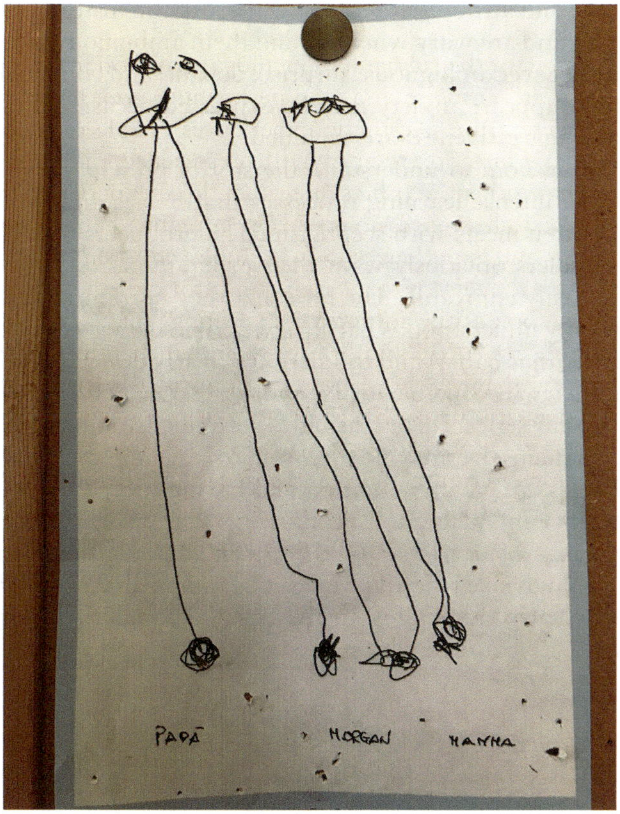

Figure 4.4 Scale: Three-year-old's view of people. Drawing: Morgan Bazalgette.

therefore fascinating to most children although, obviously, children are not all the same. One feature of moving-image media may catch some children's attention while others ignore it in favour of something different. Those that are most likely to catch a baby's attention, when she sees a TV programme or video for the first time, are the expressions and movements of human figures. In animations – far more common than live action in "baby TV" – heads and eyes are often hugely exaggerated. This stylistic feature is calculated to attract babies because facial expressions are what they encounter most frequently, and are likely to be what they soon find most meaningful. Of course, they remain meaningful to us all throughout life: other people's facial expressions – and often their eye directions as well – are the important signals from which we may judge their attitudes to us, develop our attitudes to them, or get alerted to things in the environment that we hadn't noticed. As social beings, most of us are good at judging other people's emotional states and their intentions, moods, and attitudes towards us. We respond instinctively to friendliness or hostility, and are wary when we find them ambiguous. In baby TV, emotional states are never ambiguous: surprise, delight, and convivial joy are those most likely to appear; anxiety may be expressed occasionally, but briefly; anger, fear, and aggressiveness are excluded.

My claim that learning *how* to understand the stories presented in moving images is one of the intense learning processes that babies and toddlers willingly plunge into, often meets with scepticism. The producers of TV and video for babies or toddlers obviously want their programmes to be immediately attractive and easily enjoyable. The idea that they need to be studied closely in order to be fully understood is hardly a welcome selling-point, even though this is something that babies and toddlers are clearly doing, especially when they insist on re-viewing one particular short video or episode, or are dedicated to one particular series. Unsurprisingly, the audience studies undertaken by the producers themselves pay no attention to learning: they want to be sure that their viewers are paying attention and having fun. Several years ago, I interviewed the person at Ragdoll Productions who was in charge of organising group viewings of *In the Night Garden* in contexts such as nurseries, and videoing the audience reactions. In every example that she showed me, the children were clearly enjoying what they saw – though they were of course older than the 0–2-year-olds who make up a substantial part of that show's audience.

A much more intensive type of research is done by Moonbug, the company that makes *Cocomelon*. David Segal's description of this in the *New York Times* was based on what he had observed in Moonbug's London headquarters:

> Sitting on a sofa in a glass-walled room, a 2-year-old in a blue T-shirt is riveted by an episode of *Cocomelon*, an animated cartoon series full of vivid colors, cherubic children and earworm songs like "Miss Polly Had a Dolly" and "Ten Little Duckies." Three adults stand outside a closed door, watching the toddler watch the television. One studies a computer screen that shows a live feed from a camera pointed at the tyke.
>
> It's audience research day at Moonbug Entertainment, the London company that produces 29 of the most popular online kids' shows in the world, found on more than 150 platforms in 32 languages — and with 7.8 billion views on YouTube in March alone. Once a month, children are brought here, one at a time, and shown a handful of episodes to figure out exactly which parts of the shows are engaging and which are tuned out.
>
> (Segal, 2022)

I am somewhat surprised that Moonbug is able to find 12 different two-year-olds every year who are each prepared to sit on their own in a strange room and watch *Cocomelon* – especially given that many of them (like Sunu in Chapter 1) would have started watching it by the age of four months – but Segal's report seems reliable and is supported by photographs. Segal says that the research doesn't merely consist of observing the child's interest in *Cocomelon*: as well as the main screen that the toddler is watching, there is another smaller one, "that plays a continuous loop of banal, real-world scenes – a guy pouring a cup of coffee, someone getting a haircut – each lasting about 20 seconds." What the researchers have to note is how often, and at what points in the *Cocomelon* episode, the toddler's interest is caught by the other screen. That will, they believe, indicate which bits of the episode are failing to hold the child's attention.

This is the kind of research that is vilified by the www.raisewildflowers.com website that I discuss in Chapter 3. It presents as deeply sinister the fact that shows such as Moonbug's are "carefully designed to hold a young child's attention" and therefore "act as a drug, a stimulant." The only thing that I find surprising about the Moonbug research is that they think a two-year-old will only look at 20-second clips of coffee-pouring and haircutting scenes if they're not completely riveted by *Cocomelon*. Since most toddlers know that hot coffee and sharp scissors are both very dangerous, and they may also be interested in live-action videos involving adults, since they rarely see them, I would have thought they would at least be intrigued by what the Moonbug team optimistically calls The Distractatron.

However, it does seem that *Cocomelon* does successfully hold babies' and toddlers' attention. Segal points out that it has 134 million YouTube subscribers and was watched for a total of 33 billion minutes in 2021. Predictably, his article generated 101 comments in the *New York Times*, the majority of which were clearly not from the audience sectors that Segal's statistics represent. Most were savagely negative about TV in general and/or *Cocomelon* itself. Many were also keen to boast of alternative activities such as "reading lots of library books, swimming, walking the dog, going to the park, sledding, gardening, cooking together": good indicators of the *New York Times*' readership (71% white, 93% college or university-educated). A similar reader explained the advantages of not watching TV at all: "We did it. Books, games, legos [sic], crayons, markers, music. Kid paid attention in school. By the way was reading 4–5th grade books in first grade. Went to top 7 university." These comments remind me of Colwyn Trevarthen's concern about the goal-driven learning that American academics seemed to be prioritising, which I quote in Chapter 2.

Over their first few weeks, babies' curiosity about the people and things they see around them becomes ever more intense. It is widely believed that the only possible value of moving image material for babies and toddlers is whether it can teach them what are generally assumed to be the most accessible and useful categories of knowledge that children in the 0–3 age-group should be acquiring: language, letters, numbers, and colours. I am saddened by this preoccupation with learning targets that are supposed to enable your child to "get ahead" before she enters preschool. It neglects the far wider range of learning that children in these four vital years eagerly try to undertake. In the next five chapters, I describe the roles of TV and video-viewing in the lives of what I'd rather call "the amazing twos."

TAKEAWAYS

Further reading on human development

Ghosh, A. (2021). *The nutmeg's curse: Parables for a planet in crisis*. John Murray.

Graeber, D., & Wengrow, D. (2022). *The dawn of everything: A new history of humanity*. Penguin.

Mithen, S. (2004). *After the ice: A global human history*. Orion Books.

An online search for *obstetric dilemma hypothesis* will lead you to the current debates about this idea, scholarly articles, and diagrams illustrating how the pelvis changed shape.

An online search for answers to a question such as *Do the Brits hate children?* leads to a huge range of debates and speculations from social media such as Mumsnet and Reddit, and from broadsheet newspapers and public service TV channels.

References

Davis, J. T. M., & Hines, M. (2020). How large are gender differences in toy preferences? A systematicreview and meta-analysis of toy preference research. *Archives of Sexual Behaviour* (49). doi.org/10.1007/s10508-019-01624

Laudicina, N. M., & Cartmill, M. (2023). Clavicle length and shoulder breadth in hominoid evolution. *The Anatomical Record (Hoboken), 306*(8), 2090–2101. doi.org/10.1002/ar.25144

Lepore, J. (1998). *The name of war: King Philip's war and the origins of American identity*. New York: Vintage.

Sanghera, S. (2021). *Empireland*. Dublin: Penguin Books.

Segal, D. (2022, May 8, 2022). A kids' show juggernaut that leaves nothing to chance. *New York Times*. Retrieved from www.nytimes.com/2022/05/05/arts/television/cocomelon-moonbug-entertainment.html?unlocked_article_code=1.5k8.Pa5_.F0bcLYskJQLI&smid=url-share

Chapter 5

Essential elements of narrative, and why they're important

The first sentence of Alfie's that I recognised was performed in public when he was about seven months old. He was being held in someone else's arms in the hallway of their house at the end of a social gathering, just after one of the guest families had left. He told a very simple story, in response to someone mentioning another baby's name, by presenting a sequence of three very clear Makaton signs: "baby" – "gone" – "home." It was a lovely moment, illustrating how simple sign language can enable a very young child to communicate information to others and begin to be seen as a member of a social group. It contributes to their becoming part of their family's and community's cultures very early in life. Obviously this happened too quickly for me to take a photo, but Barry Ecuyer has imagined it beautifully (See Figure 5.1).

The twins had been using Makaton for some time, taught to them by Phoebe, who had learned the sign language when she worked in a school for children with autism. When the twins were able to sit up in high chairs for their meals, the signs for "finished," "more," "stop" – and of course "no" – quickly became useful. Learning them was reinforced by watching the entertainer Justin Fletcher, whose show *Something Special* has been broadcast in the BBC channel CBeebies since 2003, and is now available on iPlayer and YouTube Kids. It is designed to introduce children to Makaton signing and is aimed primarily at those with delayed learning and communication difficulties, so Phoebe was already familiar with it for professional reasons. But it was very useful before the twins could communicate with speech. They enjoyed it, loved Fletcher's "Mr Tumble" character, and soon learned more signs, continuing to use them until their speech was well-developed. But as Alfie's statement had shown, long before that, even Makaton provides a way in to sharing information and providing explanations: essential functions of language and for bonding with others.

Charles Darwin's book *On the Origin of Species by Means of Natural Selection* (whose subtitle, *Preservation of Favoured Races in the Struggle for Life*, now tends to get less publicity) was published in November 1859. Its contradiction of religious creation myths was initially received with much horror and derision but before long, scientific investigations inspired by the

DOI: 10.4324/9781003751236-6

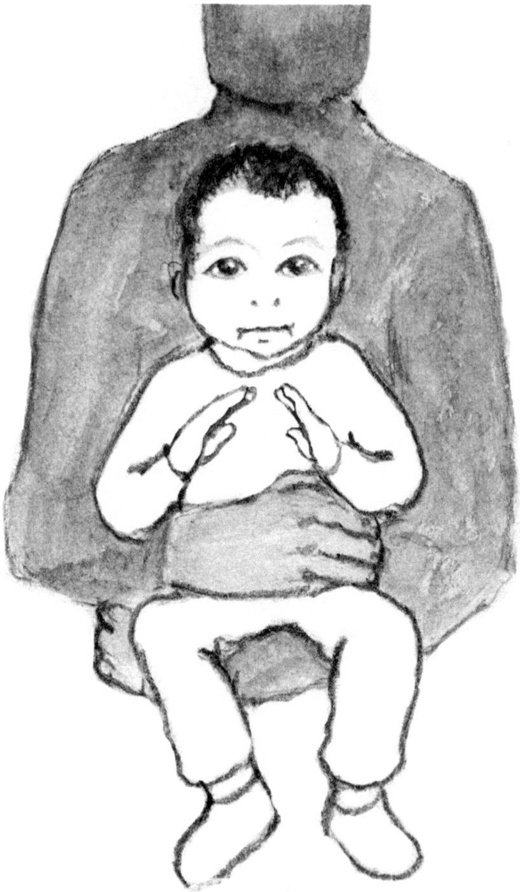

Figure 5.1 Making the Makaton sign for "home."

concept of evolution began, and have continued to proliferate ever since. And once people had stopped believing that language began with Adam and Eve in the Garden of Eden, one of the many questions that began to be asked was "when DID language begin?." There is fossil evidence in skeletons from at least two million years ago that proves pre-humans' physical capacity for making sounds with the voice. But theories vary widely on when and how spoken language actually developed: some say two million years ago, others think it could be as recent as 200,000 years ago. There is at least some agreement that it must have always been a social phenomenon, and that perhaps it appeared in different places and at different times. I like Michael Tomasello's theory that language must have begun to develop – or at least was strongly fostered – in hunting and foraging groups, where it would have been essential for everyone to maintain awareness of where all the others were and what they were doing: eye contact and gestures would have been useful, especially when silence was necessary, but being able to exchange at least a few noises, if not what we would call "words," would have been even more effective. At the same time, planning ahead must also have developed, involving the sharing of information and remembering agreements. Another human activity that always needs vocal communication is when someone is lost.

The lost person or group needs to try and let others know where they are. Equally, those others need to try and attract the lost one's attention and reassure them that help is on the way. But there are other collaborative activities that require a communication form that's more expressive, as well as more complex, than gesture and eye direction: making tools, constructing shelters, and inventing traps for wildlife such as the huge and elaborate "desert kite" structures in the Sahara, which reveal knowledge of herd behaviour and thus the ability to agree and design a way to trick animals into running to their deaths.

It isn't possible to pin down exactly when more complex languages developed. In any case, they probably started to emerge in more than one place, at different times and maybe also in different environments. We can all think of many situations where spoken language is really needed (especially as we reach for our phones!) such as catching up with a friend or relation, making a plan, borrowing something (and explaining that we'll give it back), sharing important news – and many more. But we can't know that much about what ancient societies needed to talk about.

We can however be sure that a very important part of language use, as it developed, must have been story-telling. Again, stories could have arisen long before language: initially in urgent requirements for essential information, and later being expressed through mime, dance, and music – starting perhaps as drumming and wordless vocals. We can at least make some guesses about ancient stories. For example, about 51,200 years ago in a cave on the

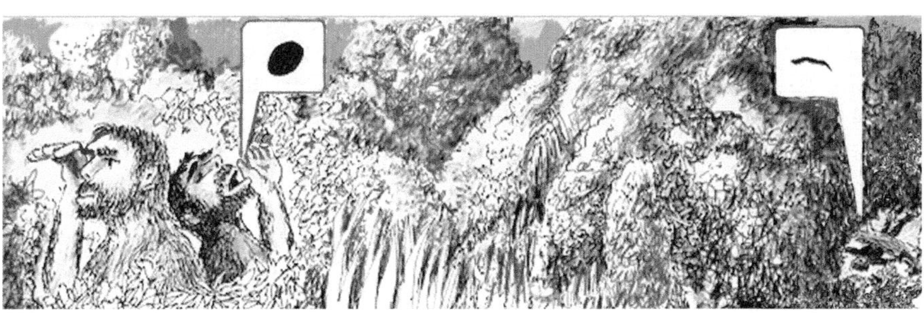

Figure 5.2 "Lost."

island of Sulawesi (Indonesia), some people made a painting in red ochre on a cave wall, which shows human figures facing a huge wild pig, in what could be a hunting scene (Ghosh, 2024). As it is an action image, it almost automatically generates questions and speculation, such as "what will happen next? Will they kill the pig? Will the pig kill one or more of them? Are some already wounded?" In other words, it sets up the essential elements of narrative. Although "narrative" is often used to mean the same as "story," I'm using it here in its broader sense of "an account of connected events" and will also hold on to the idea that it can refer to the *ways* in which a story can be structured and presented. There are actions happening in the Indonesian cave image, there are protagonists, we can see possibilities, and we're not going to see how the story plays out. But we could, if we wanted to, invent a story to go with it, and tell it in mime, spoken language or song – or all three!

Stories are an ancient and essential part of human culture. They range from the extremely simple, like Alfie's explanation of where the baby had gone, to elaborate, never-ending sagas such as *Coronation Street* (British TV series, started in 1960). We all tell stories, perhaps every day. Even if we just want to present brief information like "Sorry I'm late but I missed the bus" we have created a tiny "story," since that little utterance includes four causally interlinked elements: I missed the bus, which has made me late, and because of the effect on your plans, I'm sorry. Funny stories, juicy gossip, or dramas like the one that I couldn't resist telling to at least four different people the week before I wrote this (caught in a storm: falling masonry: narrow escape) – these are all vital and often pleasurable parts of most people's social lives.

In large modern cultures, narrative has an important role, and not just in fiction. News stories not only offer contexts, causes, and effects of incidents and policies, but generate speculation and divide opinions (and, yes, are sometimes not actually true). Within our own social and professional contexts, we exchange accounts of events and experiences, discussing motivations, responses, implications, exploring possibilities for subsequent actions or events, expressing emotional reactions, or deriding foolish behaviour. Some use social media to share untrue stories in order to generate prejudices and hate. Most of us are curious, at least sometimes, about why something happened the way it did (or did it really?), and about what caused a person or group to act in a certain way. And most of us are anxious to get at the truth, even those who just want to find, or perhaps invent "evidence" to support a particular belief and may construct narratives to attack an assumed consensus: the far-right insistence on "dangers" presented by asylum-seekers is unfortunately a familiar example of invented threats. In a broader sense however, narratives help us to structure and explain much of our everyday experience. They are also part of how we speculate about the past. Reflecting on how something came about, or how it played out, may affect how we behave in certain situations. It can be a way of helping to make sense of things, and it can generate long-term frames of mind that can be either pessimistic or optimistic. Most belief systems, especially religions, are based on founding narratives or legends.

What happened? Why did it happen? What happened next? What might be the result? These are questions that relate to natural phenomena as well as human activities (both, in the case of falling masonry). And of course, they are also questions that structure the way we think about our own experiences, as well as the way we imagine things that might happen – which for some of us can expand into the stories that we ourselves invent. Narratives get repeated, passed on from person to person, group to group, and from generation to generation, evolving as they go. Parents tell their children about events from their own childhood, as well as reminding them of what they were like when they were little. Maintaining a sense of the past and our links to it is an important part of both individual and group identities.

It is important to understand and appreciate how early in life the sense of narrative starts to develop. For a long time, it was believed that babies and toddlers live in a "here and now" world and can't think about the past. In the late 1970s and early 1980s, new research methods established that even nine-month-olds are beginning to be able to remember things. In 2004, Patricia Bauer provided a detailed explanation of how neuroscientific methods have continued to produce more evidence about the early development of memory (Bauer, 2004). However, simply remembering an event is only part of how the ability to tell stories develops. We usually also need to remember, and maybe discuss with others, why something happened and probably also what the result was. Hood and Bloom's 1979 study was an important step forward in overturning the earlier consensus that children's ideas about cause and effect don't start to develop until they are older than four (Hood et al., 1979). Their detailed and painstaking research method contrasts with the many surveys that I described in Chapter 2. They carried out an initial observational study of two children's play and language, starting when they were about 16 months old. Then they spent 17 months in individual home visits with them and with six other children. Each visit was with the child's parent always present, recording family conversations and analysing samples of it, starting when the children first began using "causal" words (such as "because," "so," and "why") as well as anything they said after an adult posed a question that included words such as "how" or "why." This is important learning for many reasons. It not only starts to establish children's understanding of the world: for example, why certain actions or events may always have bad, or good, results. On a simple everyday level, it's learning that parents and carers constantly strive to impart, for example "you could hurt your brother if you push him like that!"

My own research method was similar to Hood and Bloom's in some ways: it was based in the home, used observation, and collected recordings for analysis. In their *Developmental Review* article, Hood and Bloom explain extensively the very complex and lengthy processes of analysing all these data, the criteria they used, and their very detailed findings: I will not attempt to summarise them here. Before their study was published, it was the work of Piaget, published between 1925 and 1972, that had constituted the standard opinion on children's understanding of causality. This claimed that until the age of 7 or 8, children could not have any concept of one event causing another: they could know that they were juxtaposed in time, but couldn't understand the relationship between them. Hood and Bloom demolished this belief, providing ample evidence of the children's causal statements, which used the words "because" (usually abbreviated as "cos") or "so" to connect two events, for example as in "I don't want to, cos I'm too tired" and "that gate is in the doorway so the baby can't get into the kitchen."

I have written about Hood and Bloom's research at some length for two reasons. Firstly, because understanding causality is such a vital element of human thought, dialogue, and decision making, not only in everyday life, but also in larger, and ultimately much more significant contexts: ethics, law, and politics. And secondly, because it is also the essential "driver" of narratives. It is the basis of the desire to discover why something happened, or to find out what actions, or changes of circumstance, will or could be caused by a particular event, action, or set of circumstances. We know there are links between cause and effect – but in each case, it's the desire to find out the cause(es) that sparks our curiosity. And causes are central to narrative. They explain why something happened, perhaps bringing in their wake a series of prior events that led to the main cause; and they can be a key factor in grabbing our attention: "why ever did that happen?" and "whose fault was it?" Narratives may start with the actions, states of mind, or conditions that lead up to an event. *Hamlet* is one example: in Scene 1, Hamlet finds out that his father has not died naturally but was murdered, and the rest of the play is about how he finally gets round to doing something about it. Some other narratives start with an event such as a murder, and the story is about discovering the cause: many detective stories follow that structure.

Unsurprisingly, many moving image stories for babies and toddlers have a much simpler structure: either it's a problem which is quickly resolved, or it's an instructional presentation thinly disguised as fun. For example, browsing dozens of short videos for toddlers on YouTube Kids, I identified four common story structures:

- Different needs or preferences of older and younger siblings are resolved through kindness on the part of the older one.

- A child or a group of children need to learn some numbers, or the names of different colours.
- Something surprising or a bit frightening turns out to be completely harmless, or even nice/desirable.
- A child learns how to use a toilet and why it's important to flush it afterwards.

A large number of the YouTube videos for babies and toddlers are versions of nursery rhymes or popular songs – although of course many of those are also stories. What is noticeable however – for British families at least – is that virtually all the videos on YouTube Kids have strikingly similar stylistic features. Characters always have big eyes and heads. Voices, music, and movement are all loud and rapidly changing, colours are bright, and settings often complex. While it can be argued that these features are not individually objectionable, the similarities across dozens of different series seem wearily predictable and potentially boring. A few begin with a human presenter, in a state of extreme excitement, facing the viewer, singing a song, or uttering a greeting (as shown in Chapter 8, children younger than six may not understand that presenters are *pretending* to be talking to them!).

We grownups have basic expectations of any narrative that we choose to read, watch, or listen to. For most of us, these are probably three: that it should stimulate curiosity, meet the need to discover causes and consequences, and arrive at satisfying, but also, if possible, unexpected conclusions. So narrative enjoyment has a lot to do with our emotions. We are used to thinking of emotions in terms of the six that get listed in response to any online search: happiness (or joy), anger, fear, sadness, disgust, and surprise (some also include contempt, though love and hate, for some reason, are rarely included) However, the Estonian neuroscientist Jaak Panksepp's research on the evolution of neural systems identified four basic emotions: fear, panic, rage, and "seeking," which remain embedded in what he calls "the ancient circuits" of our brains, because they would have been essential for the survival of pre-humans. To call "seeking" an emotion may seem strange. Panksepp uses that term to cover feelings of engagement and excitement: the feelings that generate curiosity, anticipation, and investigation, and, he claims, it helps to "cement the perception of causal connections in the world and thereby creates ideas" (Panksepp, 2004). So we could say that "seeking" is the emotion that drives us to go on watching or to continue turning the pages, not "passivity" or "addiction" (see also Chapter 6).

In an earlier paper, Panksepp and Bernatzsky had suggested that "seeking" could be associated with the efforts we make in following the rhythms and sounds of music (Panksepp & Bernatzsky, 2002). Music, such as an adult's singing or humming a tune, is one of the types of sound that babies probably hear before birth. But in their early weeks of life, hearing it directly from a parent or other close family member or friend, as they are cuddled to settle them down for sleep, or for reassurance after being distressed, is different. It's an early and important way of starting to discover the world they have been born into: gentle, resonant sounds organised into rhythm, sequence, and variation, perhaps becoming familiar through repetition as the days go by. It is also, inevitably, translated into more "help your child get ahead" propaganda for parents, as in the UNICEF "baby music" advice ("Baby music: The soundtrack to your child's development," 2022) and numerous online offers such as "Music for Babies' Brain Development," "Sleep Instantly Within 3 Minutes," "Soothing Lullaby Music" (and 46 others in the search I just did). Music is perhaps humanity's most ancient and wonderful cultural form, which probably started to develop before language: it is depressing to see it reduced to the function of a pacifier.

Many months before they learn to speak, as well as in the later months before they are born, babies are likely to be experiencing music's aural patterns of rhythm and repetition, as well as the features of the speech that they can hear, whether overheard or, once they are born, spoken directly to them. In song and speech, as well as in instrumental music, they will be starting to recognise different rhythms, repeated patterns of sound, and to notice variations, for example, between soft and soothing utterances and harsh or irritated exclamations, long before these become really meaningful. In their article "The Human Nature of Music" (Malloch & Trevarthen, 2018), Malloch and Trevarthen argue that "music is at the centre of what it means to be human – it is the sounds of human bodies and minds moving in creative, story-making ways." They describe case studies, based on the principles that "any attempt to understand how human life has evolved its unique cultural habits needs to start with observing what infants know and can do" and that "our innate communicative musicality is the 'raw material' for cultural forms of music and the rules of grammar and syntax." Starting with images of new-borns responding to adult expressions, movements, and sounds with their own movements and gaze, they describe case studies that demonstrate how infants are "born ready to interact and discover [their] musical culture."

There is a vast academic literature on the different ways that people listen to music, much of it discussing the different ways in which people in various cultures respond to music.

We all know that music can evoke emotional responses and memories. It can remind us of places, people, and events. And because it is a time-based art form, the experience of listening to music can feel like the experience of a story unfolding – and of course many songs – especially nursery rhymes – do tell a story. Once babies start watching TV, they may (as many of us do) start to think of specific characters or events from a series when they hear its theme tune. Some people may imagine a story alongside music they are listening to; others may link it to the memory of an event, re-telling it to themselves as they listen. It is unlikely that we will ever be able to find out what babies think about as they start to hear music, but we can at least see their responses: waving arms and legs, smiling, etc. – or maybe just relaxing and going to sleep – and of course we encourage their responses when we play them some music, and when we hum or sing to them. So music can be seen as a significant aspect of some narratives, even at its most basic level of generating and guiding our responses to a story. Susan Young's book, *Music in Early Childhood*, is a valuable handbook for those who want to develop ways of including music in Early Years settings (Young, 2024).

Narrative matters a lot, in the sense that it is bound up with our experiences, both daily and life-long. It explores, and often explains, cause and effect, motivation, and emotional states such as curiosity, sadness, fear, suspense, joy, love, amusement, and communality. As babies start to follow the very simple narratives of picture books, baby videos and TV series, they gradually become able to relate them to the events, relationships, and emotions that they are experiencing in real life. As they grow up, narratives – and how they think about them – will contribute (for good or ill) to their moral judgments, relationships, life choices, and political beliefs. Some may be writing stories, performing on stage, or making films. But they will all also use narrative in their everyday lives, whether sharing experiences, explaining how and why something happened, or supporting an argument. Their own and others' narratives will be a crucial part of building their sense of community and shared cultures.

TAKEAWAYS

Further reading

Panksepp, J. (2004). *Affective neuroscience.* Oxford: Oxford University Press.

Young, S. (2024). *Music in early childhood: Exploring the theories, philosophies and practices.* London: Routledge.

Observation

When watching TV with child/ren, look for moments when they are reacting to an event in a story. If they are upset by it, you should decide whether to pause the programme then or to wait till the end, when you could invite their interpretations, rather than imposing yours, for example "Ooh, I wonder why he did that?" See also Chapters 7 and 8. Respond encouragingly to a child's comments, and take opportunities to explore questions such as what the results of a particular action or event might be, for example, what might happen next, or how another character might react.

The Babysong project was established by the Froebel Institute and Canterbury Christchurch University: it worked with Early Years practitioners to explore ways in which singing and song can be incorporated into day-care settings. It offers a number of strategies for musical activity with babies, such as mirroring their vocalisations, humming softly when holding a baby, and matching sounds to actions. The resulting *Babysong Booklet* is downloadable from www.ragdollfoundation.org.uk/wp-content/uploads/2017/01/BabysongBooklet_CCCU_Feb2017.pdf

References

Baby music: The soundtrack to your child's development. (2022). Retrieved from www.unicef.org/romania/stories/baby-music-soundtrack-your-childs-development

Bauer, P. (2004). Getting explicit memory off the ground: Steps toward construction of a neuro-developmental account of changes in the first two years of life. *Developmental Review*, *44*(6), 347–373.

Ghosh, P. (2024). *World's oldest cave art found showing humans and pig*. Retrieved from: www.bbc.co.uk/news/articles/c0vewjq4dxwo

Hood, L., Bloom, L., & Brainerd, C. J. (1979). What, when and how about why: A longitudinal study of early expressions of causality. *Monographs of the Society for Research in Child Development, 44*(6).

Malloch, S., & Trevarthen, C. (2018). The human nature of music. *Frontiers in Psychology, 9*.

Panksepp, J. (2004). *Affective neuroscience*. Oxford: Oxford University Press.

Panksepp, J., & Bernatzsky, G. (2002). Emotional sounds and the brain: The neuro-affective foundations of musical appreciation. *Behavioral Processes, 60*(2), 133–155.

Young, S. (2024). *Music in early childhood: Exploring the theories, philosophies and practices*. London: Routledge.

Chapter 6

Four types of viewing behaviour, and why parents needn't worry

In Chapter 2, I discussed the negative terms that many researchers have used to refer to children's TV-viewing, such as "exposure" and "use." The four terms I discuss in this chapter – "passive," "mesmerised," "staring," and "addiction" – get used by some people, including some parents and grandparents, as a disparaging way of referring to babies' and toddlers' TV-viewing behaviour, labelling it as at least time-wasting, but also possibly dangerous. In this chapter, I bring my own video-based research method to the fore in order to demonstrate how we can think about their viewing in a different way. Researchers rarely refer to the types of intense and minute observations that were the basis of my research, and very few researchers have studied their own families' relationships with moving image media as extensively I did. The classic parental studies of babies and toddlers by, for example, Piaget and Darwin, are useful precedents although of course they didn't address, or use, moving image technologies. The "Further reading" section in the "TAKEAWAYS" at the end of this chapter offer an academic paper discussing the potential conflicts of interest that could affect such studies.

But first, a brief discussion of parental attitudes to TV- and VOD-viewing. There are plenty of parents who enjoy these media themselves, are clued-up about them, and who like to exchange opinions with other parents about what they think children enjoy viewing. Such discussions are much in evidence on UK-based sites such as Mumsnet, where the Telly Addicts group discusses the qualities of different TV shows, and their appropriateness for different age-groups. Reddit.com has also had many postings and discussions on how parents manage TV with babies and toddlers. Nevertheless, in the offline, face-to-face world, there are also parents who have read or heard about the alleged dangers of babies' and toddlers' TV-watching and, maybe particularly if they don't like TV much themselves, feel strongly that these are real dangers. And there are many grandparents and well-meaning friends who tend to stoke up parental anxieties about whether their children should be watching TV, referring to the millions of online search results that quote "science" and "research findings" and "official advice" that tell them they shouldn't. So it's not surprising that a lot of parents feel anxious about their

DOI: 10.4324/9781003751236-7

children's relationships with TV, and many use one or more of this chapter's four terms, either actually to disparage their children's viewing behaviour, or simply because they feel it's a generally acceptable way to describe it. But some feel unhappy about the quandary that all these conflicting arguments have created for them.

One Reddit thread that I found was started by a mother justifying her decision to allow her 11-week-old daughter to watch *Dory's Reef Cam* (Disney Plus 2020) by pointing out that "she's laughing, making noises and just generally really enjoying herself." Like all parents, she was alert to the sounds her baby made and could confidently recognise the signs of happiness: as long as she could hear them, she wasn't going to worry. But her post generated many responses and discussions of "screen time." A little later in the same thread, another parent said "… they might seem like they 'like it' because they stare at it" which she linked to the fact that much of what they watch "seems designed to hypnotise a child." Judging by this – and by her later comment on herself "staring at Instagram" – she'd been looking at www.raisewildflowers.com or something similar (see my objections to this in Chapter 3).

"Staring" is commonly used by people who object to TV for children and want to negatively characterise a child's viewing behaviour. But in the adult world, many of us may say "staring" self-deprecatingly but light-heartedly, for example, when describing how we flop out in front of the TV at the end of a busy day, or condescendingly when characterising the behaviour of the people we've seen looking at their phones on a bus or a train. It's a word which is not associated with close attention or interpretation. It implies an absence of thought – we often use the term "just staring" with the implication that whoever is just staring is not engaging with, or reacting to, the thing(s) they are staring at. So people don't usually refer to audiences "staring at an opera," an intent reader "staring at a book," or an art enthusiast going to a gallery to "stare at the pictures." Saying that someone is staring implies that they are not really paying much attention to what they see and aren't exercising any critical effort: in fact, maybe not thinking at all. However, we may use the same term to express someone's amazement or shock: "he just stood there staring at the crash!"

The Reddit contributor's expression could have been spoken as "they might *seem* like they 'like it' " which would have been intended as a way of warning parents that when they see a child staring at the TV, they shouldn't assume that she likes what she is watching, or that it is good for her. However, that particular contributor was clearly not "anti-TV" herself, since she – and her child/ren – were *Bluey* fans (see Chapter 10 for more about *Bluey*). She would have been able to judge her children's enjoyment of *Bluey* because much of it is comedy and, like a lot of comedies, demands a certain amount of social/cultural belief, like "Dads always make mistakes when they do the housework." So I suppose the reason that this parent put the words "like it" in quote marks, and implied that other parents who use that term are a bit

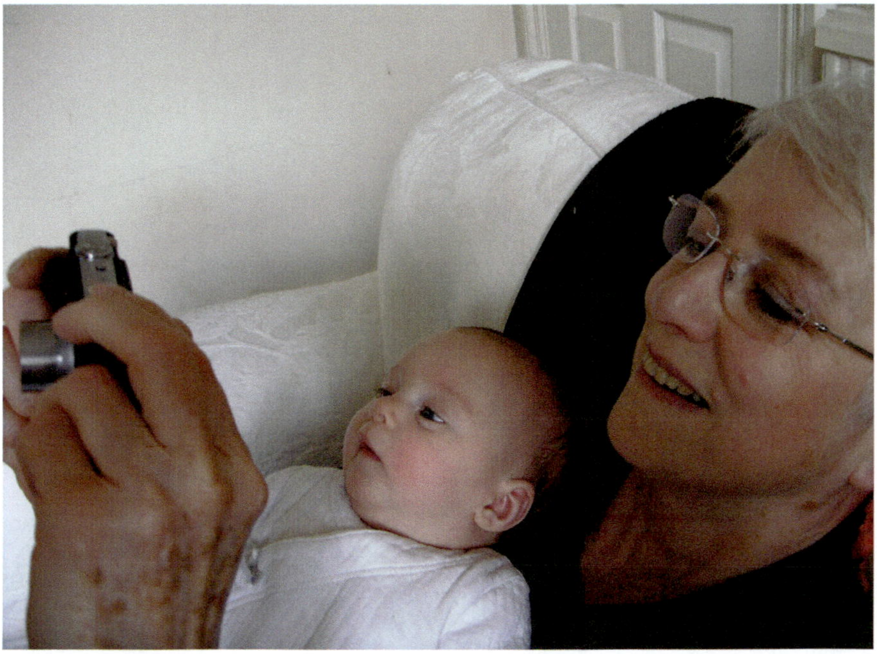

Figure 6.1 Connie at eight weeks, studying camera images. Photo: Phoebe Bazalgette.

naïve, is that she classifies "she likes it" as a rather feeble response. Or, as a parent of what must be at least toddlers, not babies, she may just think that any parent who believes that an 11-week-old is capable of "liking" anything on TV is obviously deluded. Eleven weeks is, however, only one week short of the age by which the majority of babies in the Sheffield University study I referred to in the" Introduction" (and my own grandchildren) were established TV and VOD viewers.

If all these terms can be no more than a rather vague or unreliable judgment about a pre-verbal child's reaction to a programme or a video, what kinds of positive judgment can we make? Do we need to see obvious responses such as laughter or comments? Or could we interpret "staring at the screen" as attentiveness? The babies in the following two images are certainly staring, but do they also seem to be attentive?

The Figure 6.1 photo was taken in the old days before we all had cameras in our phones, and when reviewing photos on a mobile phone screen was a less common activity. I'm shown checking through some pictures that I had just taken on my little camera, before I picked Connie up and settled on the sofa to look at them. At the moment when Phoebe took this photo, I wasn't aware of what Connie was doing. In the second image, Evie is sitting on her

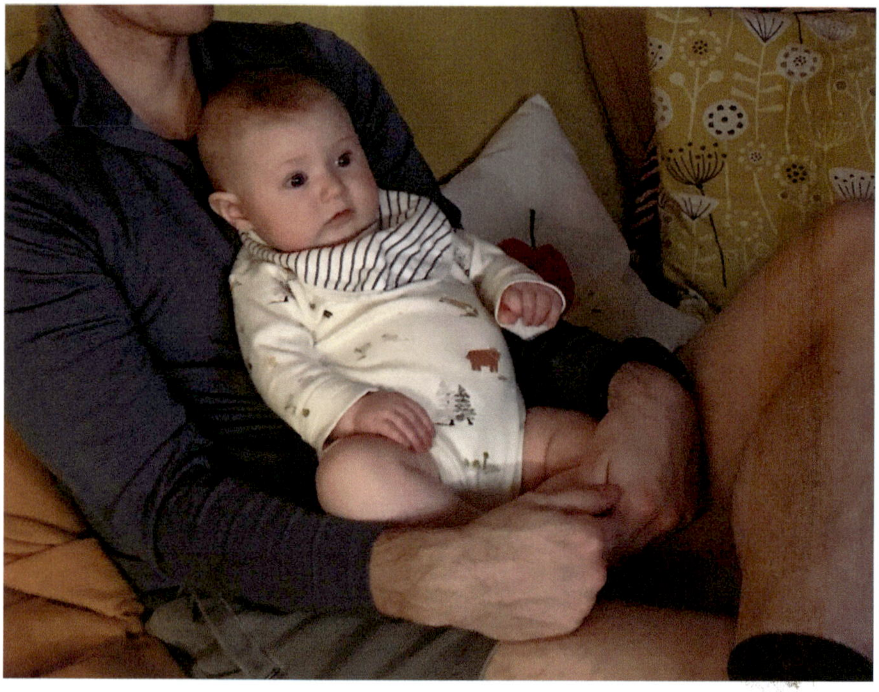

Figure 6.2 Evie at five months, watching *Moana* with her dad. Photo: Cary Bazalgette.

father's lap, quite late at night, watching *Moana* (Disney 2016) on a big TV screen. Her mother (out of shot) is sitting nearby: both parents are relaxed and enjoying the film.

I don't think that the expressions in either picture can be called "staring." In Figure 6.1, Connie can see the screen quite easily, though it's tiny and you can see that she has had to make quite an effort to see the people in the photos – who were also in the room with us at that moment, though it was probably the most interesting thing in her field of vision at that moment. But she might just have been fascinated by the way the images kept changing as I clicked through them. She seems more relaxed, despite her intent gaze: obviously she's in a comfortable position. Her jaw is relaxed and she might even be smiling a bit.

In Figure 6.2, Evie is watching an early part of the film where Moana is on a sunlit beach and huge Pacific Ocean waves are breaking on the sand. Evie's body is relaxed but her eyes are wide, intent, and perhaps seem curious. The screen, on the opposite wall, was enormous and the images are, to adult eyes at least, extremely beautiful. To Evie, they were probably unlike anything she had ever seen before. One of her hands is relaxed, resting on her leg; the other is raised, perhaps in the start of a "reaching" gesture. The photo was taken impulsively after I'd just opened the door to say goodnight: I was about to leave and didn't have a chance to go on observing her.

Intense concentration can also happen when toddlers are watching something very familiar. One of the things that can worry parents is when a toddler wants to keep on watching the same series, or even to watch the same thing over and over again. This may often be why words such as "obsessed" and "addicted" crop up often in social media, generating many random guesses by people searching for reassurance, as in these two comments from Wiz in 2014: "Children crave familiarity and comfort" and "kids are more empathetic and live more in the present than grown-ups do." But all the answers from the psychologists and childcare experts miss the most basic and plausible reason for toddlers needing to re-view things, which is that they have seen something that they partially understand, and it interests them enough to watch it again and try to understand it properly. This is no different from the reasons that any of us may want to see or read something again: it will be because we found it really interesting the first time, but didn't completely understand it, or maybe we missed a key plot development and want to check it out again. Or maybe we just loved it and want to get that buzz once more.

When toddlers view something repeatedly, they will inevitably, at the same time, develop their understanding of how moving image media create meanings. The "experts" do sometimes get close to this, when they guess that toddlers may need more than one viewing to understand a story fully, but they usually see this in terms of things that adults may sometimes struggle with, such as plot development or character motivation. They do not realise that the first time a 12-month-old sees something as "simple" as a point-of-view shot or parallel montage (see Chapter 3) they may well not understand it. But by that age they are likely to have some grasp of the narrative and are eager to go back and try again. On each viewing, they will understand a little more. I wouldn't entirely discount the responses on Wiz that I quoted earlier, but I do not believe that they explain most cases of the "repeat-viewing" phenomenon, especially when children display the "intense concentration" indicators that I have described above.

"Hypnosis," "addiction," and "obsession" are rather more anxiety-reflecting terms that are also sometimes used in relation to children's TV-watching. Adults of course also use them about their own behaviour: not just, or not necessarily, about TV-watching – though "I'm addicted to ..." is quite often used jokingly by people wanting describe their relationship with a favourite programme or series. But when they are used to characterise a child's viewing behaviour, it has to be, at least implicitly, the sign of a deliberate choice to invoke something serious: a medical condition perhaps. It sounds like a scientific diagnosis. Even when used light-heartedly, there can be an implication of disapproval or anxiety. Each of them expresses something uncontrollable: something that has "taken over" the child's mind. The mother I quoted in Chapter 1, referring to her two-year-old son watching TV "like a zombie," sounded fairly light-hearted, but to choose a word that refers to the "living dead" didn't sound merely humorous, and her delighted retraction of it a few minutes later indicated that her real opinion of his TV-viewing was a lot more positive.

When parents comment on their child finally stopping their repeat viewing of one programme or series, they usually comment that "she got tired of it" or "she doesn't like it any more." In offering a different way of thinking about children's TV-viewing, I hope to persuade parents and Early Years professionals that it is worth taking a closer interest in how babies and toddlers actually do engage with moving image media. So a more appropriate comment, that recognises the child's determination to learn, would be an expression that my daughter Phoebe invented to account for why the twins had moved on from one series to another: "they've used it up." In other words, they had got all they could out of it. The chances would be that what they next chose for repeat viewing would be something that's a bit more challenging. I discuss this further in Chapter 11.

Someone who wants to describe a child's relationship with TV or VOD and uses one or more of the four terms I've listed, is likely to be feeling at least a bit anxious about that relationship, but they might be condemnatory or even angry. As should be evident by now, my aim in this book is to counteract that anxiety or anger, not by producing another set of assertions, but simply by pointing out the motivation and value of "looking again." This isn't necessarily easy, especially for busy parents, but here are some suggestions.

As I argue in relation to Figures 1.1 and 6.2, a child's hands can be a good indicator of their level of attention. "Attention" is a very general term: it simply signifies that the person who exhibits it is very interested in what they can see and is making an effort to understand it fully. That interpretation is based on the dozens of observations I'd made during my year of observing the twins. Of course, children in general have many different ways of expressing their state of mind, but there is an enormous and very diverse amount of academic literature in psychology and non-verbal communication, as well as in diverse other fields (over 2500 journal articles!) about the significance of hand positions and body language in general, but practically nothing on hand positions as indicators of emotion: not surprisingly, as it would be very difficult to study. The research emphasis, when it is not dealing with medical issues or specific hand functions, is almost entirely on gesture. White and Givens' chapter, "The Non-verbal Language of Hands" (White & Givens, 2024) does offer a helpful background on how hands' expressions of non-verbal messages originate in very ancient neurocircuits of the brain. Our hands can therefore be very important indicators of mental states and particularly of emotions, even when they are in resting positions and we are not particularly conscious of what they are doing. So in these situations in which the hands are not in active use, the individual may nevertheless be intent on something that intrigues, fascinates, or maybe frightens them. "White-knuckle rides" is an extreme example that we're all familiar with (if only as reported by those who have actually been on one) but there are many much more subtle and transient hand positions: so many in fact that I would never attempt to classify them all, let alone interpret them, and it is likely that different children will adopt their own preferred hand positions to express particular feelings or states of mind, so there may not be much point in trying to classify them.

What I did notice in the case of the twins was that when their posture and facial expressions showed that they were interested in the series episode or short film that they were viewing, and they happened to be standing up when I observed them, they would most typically be holding on to something: primarily, I believe, to maintain their balance. Toddlers' legs are not as strong as adults', and their heads are much larger, in relation to their bodies, than adults' heads are, so standing still and maintaining a steady gaze is easier for toddlers if they can hold on to something. So a toddler standing up to view TV is likely to find something nearby to hold. If they are not standing up, they may well clench their hands or bunch their fingers together: in the Chapter 1 photo, Sunu is doing both of these.

I impulsively started videoing the twins watching TV for the first time when they were in the children's shoes department of John Lewis in Oxford Street, London: the TV screen was attached to a wall about six feet above the ground, so both of them found chairs to stand on and hold on to while they watched and I can't remember what the programme was: some series that they already knew, anyway. I only noticed their positions when I viewed the video later, and even then only gradually became aware of their decisive "viewing position" decisions when I started to make more videos of them at our house.

I describe in Chapter 3 how I first realised what my PhD research was mostly going to involve: many sessions of videoing the children's intent, focused gaze at the screen, and through close analysis, interpreting the bodily signals of concentration. Of course, it eventually included comments, expressions of preferences, and sometimes strong reactions – especially when they were saddened or scared (see Chapter 7), but the more varied responses I had anticipated rarely happened, at least when they were watching anything they hadn't seen before. New material was awarded their undivided attention. If they decided that they liked a series or short film (and there were several that they didn't like) they would start to express expectations about what was about to happen, especially on a second or third viewing – and some were viewed many more times than that: in fact it was more common for them to ask to re-view something familiar. I had a pile of DVDs containing short films that they had never seen: some of these they loved, but one or two they found sad or alarming, so were always slightly nervous when I suggested viewing something new (what they would call "one of your films"). They did sometimes however choose a film on the basis of the thumbnail images on the DVD cases, so they did see a number of non-mainstream short films, including the 5.5 minute *Animatou* (Claude Luyet, Switzerland 2007; on Vimeo at https://vimeo.com/220491211), which they watched 21 times over a three-month period, as described in Chapter 7 of my earlier book (Bazalgette, 2022).

It would be possible for someone with prior and strongly negative opinions about toddlers and TV to characterise this viewing style with one or more of the four terms that head this chapter, although I think they would have to be very fixed in those views to be able to maintain such judgments. But it is of course rare for a parent or grandparent to watch a child intently for the whole of a series episode, and even so it is hard to spot tiny quirks of posture and behaviour without being able to study a video of the viewing behaviour. It's more likely that the child will be seen as "peaceful" or – if the observer has a negative attitude to children's TV-viewing – to see it as the sort of passive, mesmerised behaviour that must indicate "addiction." I think that if I ever did see a child who actually did look "passive" or "mesmerised" as she viewed, I would be worrying about what other factors in her life might be affecting her behaviour.

TAKEAWAYS

If a parent is concerned about their child wanting to watch the same thing again and again, you could try, if it looks as though it could be appropriate, to suggest the possibility that the child may be hard at work, learning not only TO make sense of it, but learning HOW to make sense of it, and that they almost certainly don't need to worry about it. You can point out that they will move on sooner or later, and you could perhaps introduce the idea of "using it up." But if those interpretations don't seem appropriate it might be necessary to consider the family context and whether there are other factors affecting the child's viewing behaviour.

Further reading

Abernethy, E. (2021), "Conflict of roles: Enrolling one's own children in your research" provides a useful historical summary of this practice, with a discussion of its ethics and reliability. https://georgiactsa.org/_includes/documents/sections/research/rks/conflict-of-roles-enrolling-ones-own-children-in-your-research-ea-gc.pdf

De Stefano, Cristina. (2023). *The child is the teacher: A life of Maria Montessori*. New York: Other Press – in case Montessori's work is or was not part of your training: it is certainly worth considering her recognition of children's ability to concentrate, to control their own learning, and to enjoy rituals like tidying up the classroom and putting things away in the right places. De Stefano's book was published in English after I had completed my research, but I was delighted to recognise the parallels between Montessori's observations and mine.

References

Bazalgette, C. (2022). *How toddlers learn the secret language of movies*. Cham, Switzerland: Palgrave Macmillan.

White, J., & Givens, D. (2024). The nonverbal language of hands. In D. Chadee, & A. Kostic (Ed.), *Body language communication*. New York: Springer.

Chapter 7

Learning why and when to laugh, and how to deal with fear

An important dimension of 0–3s TV and video-viewing is the process of learning to understand the style and content of any film or series that they haven't seen before. This can be something that some parents may be nervous about, so they prefer to stick with "more of the same" in what they choose for their child to watch. But sooner or later they or the child will encounter something new, and be intrigued enough to stay with it, whether in the form of repeat-viewing, or to follow a series. But new things can be surprising. Sometimes the surprising element can be difficult to deal with at first. It may just seem bizarre, but it can be frightening. Experienced viewers understand generic signals, for example, the indicators that lead them to expect funny events and dialogue, or they may already know that anyway from the way that a film or series is promoted and reviewed. Toddlers take some time – and plenty of viewing experience – in developing the ability to recognise the generic signals of comic intentions. Until then they can sometimes be a bit puzzled, and sometimes they can be frightened.

Fear and laughter are more closely related than we usually think. If you have ever owned or looked after two or more kittens or puppies, you'll be familiar with their "play-fighting" activity. Although one attacks the other in an apparently aggressive way (and it can sometimes start looking serious enough for you to try and intervene), it is nevertheless obviously playful fighting, often involving melodramatically aggressive behaviour, but rarely including the actual infliction of pain. In Chapters 4 and 5, I refer to human evolution, and the potentially dangerous environments that pre-humans and early humans had to deal with, especially in their reliance on hunting and foraging, both of which inevitably involved danger. If they hadn't learned how to recognise the threats of danger and figure out ways of avoiding it, we wouldn't be here today. It's very likely that play-fighting of some sort was a significant part of early human toddlers' lives, preparing them for the shock of being attacked as well as enjoying the denouement of "it's only a game." It may be that the "peekaboo" game we all play with babies might, long ago, have been an early instance of humans "toughening up" their babies. Mummy suddenly vanishes and the baby may look alarmed, or just

DOI: 10.4324/9781003751236-8

nonplussed. Then she suddenly reappears: the baby laughs in surprise and relief – encouraged by Mummy's big smile and the warm humorous tones of her "Peekaboo!" utterance.

Many humorous games follow, in some form, using the convention of creating tension and then cancelling it by inducing laughter. But most narratives take a lot longer than a peekaboo game. If they're intended to be funny, the "creating tension" part always has to signal, in some way, that the threatened, unwelcome, and perhaps dangerous outcome will be averted in a way that will make us laugh, not only with relief but also with pleasure in the ingenuity of the story-telling. An excellent example occurs in the cyclone scene of the Buster Keaton silent film *Steamboat Bill Jr* (USA 1928). Keaton plays a gormless young man who is being pursued by two baddies who are determined to break up his relationship with the daughter of one of them. A chase sequence takes place at the same time as a cyclone is devastating the town. Bill Jr pauses for breath in the middle of a street as bits of rubbish go whirling past him in the wind. He is unaware that the entire front of the building behind him has been torn away by the cyclone and is about to fall on him. I won't spoil the story for you if you don't know it already: it suffices to explain that he is not killed and his lucky escape is startling, extremely funny, and was obviously dangerous to Keaton. Our laughter is magnified by the relief that Bill Jr is still alive, as well as by the typical Keaton trope of appearing to be completely unaware of the danger.

Alfie and Connie didn't laugh spontaneously and out loud at humour in a TV programme until they were 27 months old. They were watching the "Water" episode of *Teletubbies* (another hugely popular – and initially controversial – TV series for toddlers, first broadcast by the BBC in 1997 and subsequently in over 120 countries in 45 different languages). The story in this episode – which the twins had seen several times before – involves a big puddle of water, which three of the Teletubby characters encounter, one after another, each carefully negotiating it in a different way in order to avoid getting wet. But then the fourth Teletubby comes along on her scooter, rides straight through the puddle, and splashes all the others – to be followed by much laughter. There's a careful build-up to this denouement, which enabled the twins to anticipate it on what was perhaps their third or fourth viewing, and finally to laugh delightedly when it happened. This manifestation of spontaneous laughter in response to something on screen, long after they were able to follow a story, tells us something about the complexity of humour. It takes toddlers a while to build up expectations of a comic denouement.

Many years ago, back in the video-cassette era, I watched my other grandson, Morgan – then aged 27 months, dealing in his own way with what might have been anxiety about the intended meaning of a sequence in *Monsters, Inc.* (a film that both my children remember fondly, so all my grandchildren were first shown it at a very early age). This was in the era of the now-obsolete videocassettes and of the VCR machines on which they were played. Demonstrating his growing confidence with technology, Morgan sorted through the messy pile of unboxed videocassettes next to the VCR (this wasn't in my house!) until he found the one he wanted, presumably identifying it by the colour of the label, since he certainly couldn't read at that age. He installed it in the VCR, switched on the TV, pressed "play" on the VCR, and searched the movie until he found the bit he was after: the now-famous – and hilarious, to most of us – 2.47-minute scene where Randall uses the "scream-extractor" machine on Mike.[1] Morgan played, re-wound, and re-played the scene several times. He didn't show any distress – though he didn't laugh, either – but he was clearly interested in examining the scene closely. I do find this scene rather alarming, although the film as a whole is certainly a comedy. Randall is sinisterly slithery and vicious, Sully and Boo look terrified in their hidey-hole, Mike is scared as the big and threatening scream machine slowly advances on him, Fungus messes up the operation of the machine and is reduced to panic. But Morgan calmly viewed and re-viewed the scene several times: not laughing, but showing no signs of fear either. He had seen the film previously with his parents (see also Chapter 11 for an account of how the twins developed their own relationship with this film). He did this very deliberately and obviously needed to, but why he did it wasn't clear to me, and he (now grown-up) can't remember doing it. The scene does however combine comedy with danger, and Morgan may have been trying to understand why his parents laughed at it.

It was a fearful response by the twins that got me started on my PhD research. When the twins were 13 months old, Connie reacted with terror – and Alfie quickly joined in – to a scene in an episode of *In the Night Garden*, involving the Pontipine family (eight children and two parents of animated "peg-doll" type figures) in which the father's luxuriant black moustache suddenly detaches itself from his face and flies away, swooping all over the Night Garden accompanied by "swanee whistle" sounds, and looking rather like a big moth. I wasn't there when the twins were frightened by this scene, but I was intrigued by the fact that they had been terrified by something that is obviously (to more experienced viewers, at least) meant to be funny. I realised that the generic knowledge that is needed if one is to laugh at something bizarre, especially something like this which is clearly upsetting to the characters in the story, takes a while to develop, and 13-month-olds may not be able to realise the comic intention. So when I had become committed to the PhD project and the twins were 17 months old, I asked Phoebe if we could show it to them again and I would video what happened. I describe this in some detail in my previous book (Bazalgette, 2022); it suffices to say here that Connie recognised the scene as soon as it began and when the moustache flew away she started shrieking and Alfie froze, either in sympathy or in his own terrified response. Phoebe and I agreed to continue nevertheless, and by watching the scene through to the end from behind the sofa, the twins calmed down and were cheered up by the moustache's return and the happy ending.

Alfie began to express another kind of fear when he was about two, starting when he began to hate seeing the bathwater running down the plughole, and developing into a much more intense and long-lasting fear: he dreaded having to view the endings to any TV episode or film. This began when he was 28 months old and lasted for nearly a year. To the annoyance of any co-viewers, he quickly figured out how to turn off the TV as soon as he became aware that the ending was about to happen. He had become well-attuned to the ways in which films and TV episodes signal their endings in advance, which of course is easier in the case of series episodes, since each series tends to have its own typical way of signalling that the end is near. But Alfie clearly did not want to view any of the ways in which a TV drama can approach its conclusion: slowing down, problems resolved, characters either saying goodbye or happily reunited, the theme tune playing one last time. He presumably didn't want to re-experience the emotions that endings had previously generated in him: a sense of loss? Finality? It is hard to know, and he now doesn't remember doing it, although the rest of the family often remind him of how annoying it was. Children's TV is clearly different from drama series for older audiences, in which episodes will often close with a cliffhanger. In children's series, episodes usually end when problems are resolved and everyone is happy, indicating the imminent end, but the conventions of "story resolution" didn't make any difference to Alfie: it was the basic fact of "ending" that he found intolerable. Once he was discouraged from turning off the TV, he would get up and wait by the door, continuing to watch from a distance until the ending was imminent, and then run away.

Another and potentially quite different type of response, which might or might not have been fear, was expressed by Connie when the twins were 32 months old. I showed them the short film *A Sunny Day* (Gil Alkabetz, Germany 2008; available on YouTube). The central character of the film is the sun, first heard snoring behind some hills, under a night sky with twinkling stars. He wakes up, shakes himself, and rises up into the sky. His facial expressions (which are all we can see, as the sun obviously doesn't have a body, though this one does have some diminutive arms and hands) are highly exaggerated. We know he is male, partly by his deep, grunting, wordless voice, conceivably by his incessant desire for approval and admiration, but mainly by the fact that he grabs two clouds and slathers them over his face as shaving cream. The theme of the film is that everyone on the ground is trying to avoid him: wearing hats and sunglasses, pulling down blinds, using umbrellas at the beach: all of which makes him grunt with disappointment. But at the end of the day as he starts to slide down the sky towards the sea, huge crowds come to the shore and start taking photographs of the colourful sunset as he sinks below the horizon. He revels in the sight of the enthusiastic crowd lined up on the promenade. Alfie enjoyed the film and several times asked to see it again. I must admit that I don't find the film particularly funny, but Connie's reaction was much more extreme: she cried bitterly, screamed if I ever suggested showing it again and could never say why. It seemed unlikely to me that she was upset on the sun's behalf, given that he is not really a very sympathetic character, being full of self-importance and too fond of show-off stunts. My hunch about her response might be due to excessive grand-motherly admiration, and/or assuming too much on the basis of my own opinion of the film's style. But I did sense that perhaps she hated the over-the-top characterisation: the sun's exaggerated expressions and wildly emotional reactions to everything he sees. I quite liked its gentler satirising of typical seaside-crowd behaviour, but the children were unlikely to be aware of that aspect. It is possible that Connie just disliked the character's self-importance, but her reaction did resemble fear rather than disapproval. She screamed and even cried if I ever suggested showing it. Alfie didn't seem to share those feelings at all, and even seemed quite keen to see it again a few days later. But Connie shrieked her dissent to that idea.

In his book *The Second Year: The Emergence of Self-Awareness* (Kagan, 1981*)*, Jerome Kagan describes a development in toddlers' emotional lives that may relate to the kinds of fear that I have been describing. Some time after 18 months old, toddlers start to become very interested in *order*: in how things are arranged, where they belong, and doing things correctly. Alongside this there can be a lot of distress about clothing getting dirty, things being put in the wrong place, toys getting broken. They may like to counter their anxiety about order by organising toy animals or cars into lookalike groups, or by watching a toy train going into a tunnel and then coming safely out again. No doubt a lot of this is due to their increasing skill in speaking and listening, much of which is likely to include exchanges with parents and carers about putting things away, taking care not to break things, behaving properly, etc. And it must also relate to their growing awareness of cause and effect, generating the concept that in certain contexts, "this is how things always happen." It may be that they do not at first understand why it is supposed to be important to tidy things up, put them in the right places, and not break them, and may develop an almost superstitious anxiety about "correctness" and tidiness. Of course, there are plenty of people who enjoy ignoring these rules once they leave home or even just when they get their own room: they relish the mess and the freedom it represents! But I think that Kagan's argument could be extended to help explain toddlers' fearful reactions to what experienced viewers would see as merely amusing.

There is a sense in which the "moustache" and "sun" stories are similar, in that they both involve grotesque representations of what are normally inanimate objects. Both the moustache and the sun suddenly become alive and behave in exaggerated ways. And in both cases, it was Connie who first reacted fearfully. So it seems that she was particularly sensitive to bizarre representations, distortions of reality and "rule-breaking" behaviour, even when displayed by what are supposed to be inanimate objects. I think this may be fairly common amongst toddler viewers: I have seen social media posts that described toddlers getting similarly distressed by unexpected, fanciful, exaggerated events on screen: for example, "a pile of elephants standing on top of one another" was cited by one baffled mother whose toddler was briefly very frightened by an episode of *Baby Jake* (Irish Film Board and CBeebies, 2011).

This can be seen as closer to Kagan's theory. It is possible for children's fiction – whether on screen, in pictures or in story-books – to include fanciful figures and actions that are impossible in real life: fairies, magic cloaks of invisibility, flying horses, talking fish, giants, etc,, but usually these are introduced and explained in some way, if only by the addition of the word "magic." It could be the sudden introduction of something unexplained that can frighten some children, especially if it appears to be self-initiated and uncontrolled.

Alfie's fear of endings was different. Connie was displaying immediate responses to what was on the screen: Alfie was avoiding the emotions that he anticipated would be generated as a film or a series episode came to an end, by making sure that he didn't see the ending at all, and this applied to any ending, including those in material that was otherwise quite light-hearted. His reaction to another *In the Night Garden* episode could be interpreted as related to "endings": at age 13 months, he was very upset when Macca Pacca's little "bike" (known as the Og Pog) wasn't parked properly, and rolled away downhill. This might provide a clue to the fear of endings: a fear of irretrievable loss. This can of course be a deep fear for all of us, exemplified worst of all in the fear of a loved-one's death, so it could seem rather trivial to be so upset by a bike getting mislaid. But perhaps Alfie's fear should be thought of in terms of the underlying conclusiveness of something being ended or gone: an emotional state that becomes sadder as we get older and more aware of what might be – and indeed eventually will be – lost. But it is still quite a shock for a toddler experiencing "finality" for the first time. And of course the standard "they were happy ever after" is a comforting alternative.

I was interested to find that when I searched for academic studies of toddlers being frightened by something they had seen on screen, I couldn't find anything. The focus of academic work on children and fear is heavily biased – understandably – towards fear as a sign of longer-term problems such as phobias and towards the danger of children coming habitually fearful. And it would obviously be unethical to try and set up frightening events in an experimental context! But it can be alarming for parents or carers when a child suddenly becomes really frightened by something that seems innocuous. It can immediately raise fears of longer-term psychotic problems. There is also a commonly shared perception that fear is bad and dangerous: we are quick to exclaim "Don't be frightened! Look, it's not really scary!" and similar "reassurances."

In my earlier book I describe two instances of how we dealt with the twins' sudden fears. The first was when the twins were only 22 months old and were watching the Peppa Pig episode "Sports Day" (www.youtube.com/watch?v=SyWAIvH9MHc), which includes a girls-against-boys tug-of-war competition in which the rope breaks, everybody falls over, and neither team wins, resulting in much merry laughter. Connie had been upset about this before and I was invited over to their house to watch her viewing it again. When, as predicted, she screamed (aware of me watching, so somewhat melodramatically) and wept copiously until Phoebe pulled her on to her lap and asked, "You don't like it when the rope breaks, do you?" at which Connie said "no," sniffed and stopped crying at once.

I only saw Alfie's "avoiding the ending" tactic once, when we were watching *Meg and Mog* one evening. I followed him after he had run away to the kitchen and was being comforted by Phoebe. After he had calmed down somewhat, I asked him "Is it frightening to see the ending?" His response was a huge sigh of relief and a big, breathed-out "Ye-e-e-s!" That was all it took: his fear of endings gradually diminished thereafter, because my question had respected his emotional state and did not try to belittle it.

It may seem counter-intuitive to address toddlers' fear by acknowledging the source of it directly, rather than by trying to persuade them that "it's not really frightening" or "it's not real." These may seem logical reassurances from the adult point of view, but we need to remember that by acknowledging that *their* fear is real, we can show respect for their feelings at that moment. We don't have to agree that it is frightening or even try to talk about the frightening thing, unless the child wants to. We must appreciate that a toddler can easily be shocked by seeing something for the first time that seems unjustified or inexplicable. That's a normal, human response that we all share. But many things that we're used to can be shocking to a toddler seeing them for the first time.

Feeling terrified is in itself terrifying – all the more so because at that moment it feels rational and understandable: we scream when we are convinced that the frightening thing really *is* frightening. By showing respect for a toddler's fear, we acknowledge that, at the time, it is real to them. Another time, it may be appropriate to talk about things that have seemed frightening, but not while they still feel scared. What absolutely does not work and may well make a child feel worse, is to laugh at their fear response or even just try to persuade them that "it's not frightening." Fear is always real to the person who experiences it: as a significant emotion, it has always been vital to any creatures, not just humans, in its role of warning about danger. Even just speaking in "reassuring" terms, as in "it's not really scary!" is unhelpful: it denies the child's feelings and diminishes her self-confidence. Acknowledging the fear respects the child and enables her to move on in due course without feeling foolish.

TAKEAWAYS

Parents may well worry about their children being suddenly frightened of something innocuous that they see on TV or in a video, fearing that it might be the start of a phobia or long-term trauma. Suggesting that they acknowledge the fear may help. It is best not to initiate discussion about this by asking whether their child/ren have ever been frightened by something they have watched, as this could seem alarming or perhaps intrusive. If they want to discuss it with you, it may be helpful to describe one or more of the examples from this chapter.

Further reading

Hye-Knudsen, M., & Kjeldgaard, C. (2024). First they scream, then they laugh. *Evolutionary psychology*, *22*(2). This article synthesises neurobiological, psychological, and evolutionary research on fear and humour, arguing that the two are deeply connected. https://doi.org/10.1177/14747049241258355

Kagan, J. (1981). *The second year: The emergence of self-awareness*. Harvard University Press. Includes discussion of long-term effects of fear episodes and prompts for responding to parental worries about children's fears and how they can be dealt with.

Training contexts

Students may enjoy being asked about memories of their own early fears and be interested to share them with others, leading to discussion of how they coped with them (or possibly failed to do so!) and reflecting on the nature of early and apparently irrational fears. These may or may not relate to TV-viewing: the aim would be to develop empathy with a child's fears.

Note

1 There is a useful discussion of this at: www.youtube.com/watch?v=rIH8OLT7XWA

References

Bazalgette, C. (2022). *How toddlers learn the secret language of movies*. Cham, Switzerland: Palgrave Macmillan.

Kagan, J. (1981). *The second year: The emergence of self-awareness*. Cambridge, Mass: Harvard University Press.

Chapter 8

Learning how to recognise "real" and "pretend"

Most people agree that it's important to be able to distinguish between reality and illusion. But we also think it's nice for babies and toddlers to be surrounded by still and moving image representations of the kinds of thing that do not exist in the real world: imaginary creatures, animals who can talk, people who can do magic, or fly. And at the same time, many of their toys are life-size or miniature representations of real things – bears, rabbits, babies, cars, trains. As children start learning to talk, we may use terms like "real" and "pretend" without getting drawn into complicated debates about what "real" actually means: so "real" usually just means things you can see and touch. But even this quickly gets complicated as well. Animals at the zoo are real but you can't touch them. And your child can see and touch her toy fire engine, but it's not a real fire engine. And breaking it would be "a real shame." Tigers are real, but in the book you are both looking at, they're just pictures – and your child can touch them. Wearing a hat with rabbit ears, or dressing up as a firefighter, can help her to imagine what it might be like to be a real rabbit or a firefighter, and maybe demand to be treated like one. A child watching a puppet show or a live performance can be drawn into the emotional reality of the story so that he can feel the terror or the sadness: it can be "too real." As well as acknowledging his fear, you might have to explain to him that it was "just pretend."

We know that in the early stages of exploring these fascinatingly complicated ideas, toddlers may be seen touching TV screens. Adults (and indeed some psychologists) often assume that they do this because "they think it's real." I believe that a more accurate interpretation could often be that "they want to find out *how real it is*." If you search online for information about children's understanding of reality, you are likely to find statements such as "children are often confused about the difference between reality and non-reality." I find the frequent choice of the word "confused" in this context rather patronising: why choose that instead of "unsure" or even "curious about …"? It may be because seeing toddlers as "innocent" and in need of help and protection tends to be the default view: most of us share in this to some extent. It magnifies our feelings of protectiveness towards them, and

DOI: 10.4324/9781003751236-9

our senses of horror and outrage when we hear about evidence of cruelty and abuse. It's tempting just to enjoy the endearing sight of a toddler wonderingly touching a TV screen and to interpret it as evidence of his simple naivety. But I think we should still try to recognise his intense desire to investigate, discover, and learn. And we should remember that "real" and "not real" are really complicated concepts.

In this chapter, I'll describe some of the many ways in which toddlers may examine TV screens: getting close to them, touching them, and pointing to things on the screen, and I'll add my own suggestions of what I think was probably going on in these encounters. But I'll start with a reminder about how TV itself encourages us all to believe in its "reality." For example, presenters of live or apparently live shows will often end the programme by turning to the camera and saying "see you tomorrow!" Because they make eye contact with the camera, we can enjoy their friendly familiarity as though they are really talking to us, while at the same time knowing that can't see us today, and they won't see us tomorrow!

What do little children make of this? I recorded an exchange between Phoebe and Alfie when the twins were 3.7 years old, watching a presenter on the Milkshake programme (Channel 5), a transcript and discussion of which is included in my previous book (Bazalgette, 2022). Phoebe was trying to find out what Alfie made of the presenter's direct address to camera, but Alfie immediately picked up on the exaggerated, playful tone of her questions and enthusiastically joined in with the fantasy. As a child who was attending nursery by the time of this dialogue, Alfie was familiar with the style of "adult talk" to groups of children, to the extent that it enabled him to devise an alternative interpretation of the programme's efforts to make viewers believe that they are members of the Milkshake community, and are all the subjects of the presenter's direct gaze to camera. But he had his own theory about this. He assumed that there must have been some children – in some sense "hers" – who must be "there" somewhere (later he would learn the term "off camera"), which would explain not only her style of talking but also why she kept on saying "Milkshakers," as though they were some sort of special group. It had not occurred to him that this was supposed to refer to him, *and* to lots of other children watching the same programme in many other places. This reminded me of something I discovered many years ago, when discussing a TV advertisement with a class of six-year-olds: even at that age, those children did not understand what is meant by "a television audience": that is, lots of people who don't know each other and can't see each other, watching the same TV programme in many different places all over the country. Alfie had clearly assumed that there must be some children somewhere near the presenter, and was maybe a bit frustrated that they are never shown. But at the same time, he hadn't yet picked up on the fairly sophisticated convention that we are *supposed to believe* that presenters can see us, even though they can't really, which is why even the presenters of programmes for grownups will say not only "goodbye" but also "see you tomorrow" (to which, in my churlishly literal-minded manner, I usually mutter "no you won't!").

A year earlier, I had noticed Connie (aged 2.7) being suddenly distracted from her rummaging in the toy box, by the loud and distinctive voice of David Tennant on the other side of the room saying "HALLO!" at the beginning of the Bedtime Story on the CBeebies channel. She hurried back across the room to the TV and stood close to the screen, where she could see Tennant in close-up as he told the story, and could occasionally reach out towards the toys scattered around the set. And of course, in a sense Tennant did seem to be talking directly to her, which was of course what the BBC wanted her to believe, although this belief did not extend to her thinking that she could talk back to him. She became more interested in "touching" the toys.

Touching is an essential experiment: part of learning about the world, and a crucial pathway towards distinguishing between real things and representations of real things. But one interpretation of screen-touching might simply be that it's an instinctive desire to feel the reality of the screen itself (silky, warm, very slightly soft: you can distort the image by poking your finger on the surface); and perhaps also the desire to get as close as possible to an object in the image. The concept of proximity to the screen being "bad for your eyes" dates from the days of glass TV screens and 405-line images which were unpleasantly fuzzy when seen close up. But looking closely at a modern TV screen and touching the images, constructed by millions of pixels, is fascinating. So, I didn't try to stop the twins doing it, and they never wanted to watch continuously from that distance, though they did at first want to sit close to the screen.

Thinking about the reality status of images, whether on modern screens, paintings in galleries, or on cave walls, has probably always fascinated many people. For example, archaeologists wonder about what kinds of audiences (if any) cave paintings may have had. Were the paintings believed to have magical qualities or ritual purposes? Were lights (torches or lamps) used to reveal them as part of a story or performance? Were there rules about who – if anyone – was allowed to touch them? Many paintings are on cave ceilings and could never have been touched by onlookers anyway. These questions are still the subject of speculation by archaeologists, and numerous possible answers have been suggested. But it is likely that people wanted to touch them, whether or not they were allowed to. Today, art galleries have to foil the urge that many of us have: to feel the texture of paintings and the shape of sculptures, as part of our appreciation of the artist's skill. We want to feel a sense of communion with the processes that created the artwork. It's not because we think that the subject of the painting is "really there." It's because touch is an essential part of our relationship with any real object: together with sight, it confirms the reality of the object itself: its solidity, its texture, its temperature. But of course, if art works were constantly touched by hundreds of people, they would acquire a greasy surface that would damage them: hence the rules and barriers.

So one basic explanation for why a toddler wants to touch a TV screen is that it's an instinctive thing to do. As regular viewers, most of us have forgotten what a cornucopia of images, sounds and movement it offers to anyone who has never seen it before, or never been able to get up close to it. At their own house, the TV that Connie and Alfie watched was above their head height if they were standing close to it (but see Chapter 11 for my account of them watching a scene from *Mary Poppins* on that TV). At our house, the TV was on a low trolley so at first, I worried about them watching it close to and putting their sticky fingers on the screen, so I moved a coffee table in front of it, which they delightedly climbed up on and watched in extreme close-up, making it difficult for me to video their viewing behaviour; and forgotten coffee cups or plates of toast kept being knocked to the floor. So in the end, the compromise was a big IKEA footstool, positioned near the trolley, on which they could sit and watch comfortably (see Figure 8.1).

Later, they would just stand in front of the TV and touch it whenever they wanted, which I didn't mind because by then I was interested in the "touching" phenomenon. Of course, this was an unusual arrangement because I was deliberately studying their behaviour. In the 1970s when I was a busy parent who sometimes needed to leave my children watching TV alone while I got their tea ready or answered the front door, I had the same setup as Phoebe had: the (much smaller, black-and-white) TV set was on a shelf out of their reach.

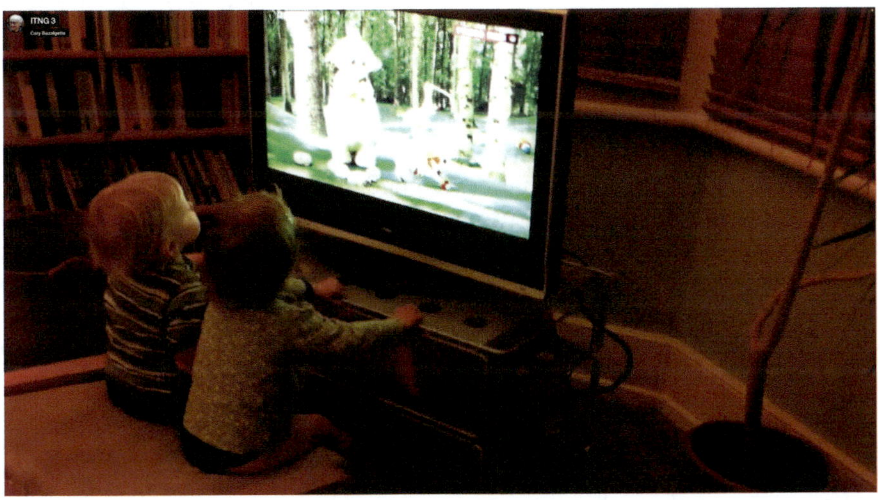

Figure 8.1 Watching *In the Night Garden*, aged 23 months. Photo by the author.

The footstool compromise for the twins meant that I was able to see when they wanted to touch the screen, and to think about why they were doing it. Although most of their viewing took place sitting with an adult on the floor or on the sofa, there were also some occasions when they chose to stand close to the screen, or would walk up to it when they wanted to point out something important to the rest of us. This would be most likely to happen when they were watching something for the second or third time and wanted to identify a particular moment that was significant for them.

While we were still in the coffee-table era and the twins were around two years old, Alfie sometimes knelt on the table to watch programmes close up, perhaps when he wanted to spot things that he especially liked. One evening he touched the beak of the toucan which is one of the "tittifer" birds in the *In the Night Garden* interludes, exclaiming "Big beak! B-I-I-G beak!" I think this was to demonstrate that he knew the words and could use them appropriately. And maybe that sometimes the word "big" just isn't big enough.

Most screen-touching before they were about 28 months was of this type: more often relating to films or programmes that they had seen before and wanted to point out to everyone else in the room. They could be seen eagerly waiting for a particular moment and then reminding the rest of us about it. The film version of the Eric Carle book *The Very Hungry Caterpillar* was a favourite: Alfie enjoyed imitating the caterpillar squirming with indigestion, and one day Connie (encouraged by Phoebe) pretended to feed it some strawberries, standing close to the screen with a bowl and a spoon. But this was not a delusion: it was clearly a performance for the other people in the room, initiated by Phoebe, in which Connie happily colluded. So what may in the very early years be a real confusion about the reality status of something on TV, this does change over time into enjoying the pleasure of ambiguous or deliberately playful representations of "reality."

I encountered a rather different "reality judgment" a few years ago. I had a 20-year-old asylum-seeker living in my house, whose escape from his home country and eventual ending-up in the UK had been complicated and often frightening, and had taken eight years. In addition to the PTSD this had left him with, it had also ensured that he had had few opportunities to watch TV, so he enjoyed watching various programmes with me. One evening I showed him an episode from one of the popular documentary-style TV series about dinosaurs (I forget which one) which began with an aerial shot of a group of CGI dinosaurs lumbering across a wide grassy plain. My guest had never seen – or even heard of – CGI before, and had left school when he was 12. So it was more or less impossible – especially in the very simple English that we had to use – to persuade him, firstly that these animals not been filmed anywhere, but had been created in a computer, and secondly, that they showed animals that haven't existed for millions of years. The skills of the CGI artists had created something that was too convincing!

Obviously, toddlers can't explain their thoughts like this, but I believe that it is safe to assume that toddlers may at least sometimes want to investigate not only what is on the screen, but also what the screen is. They do this either by getting up close or by trying to touch it. Now that they can see moving images on mobile devices as well as (or instead of) on a TV set, they are probably less likely to wonder whether what is on the screen is actually inside the TV set than 20th century children sometimes seemed to do – at least to adults who saw a child going round behind the set (if they could) and assumed that they were looking for evidence of where these people actually were. Now that we are used to moving image media, we don't realise how extraordinary it was for the 19th-century people who first saw pictures moving. Apparently, some of them did try to get behind the screen to find out what was there.

TAKEAWAYS

Further reading

Davies, M. M. (1997). *Fake, fact and fantasy: Children's interpretations of television reality*. Mahwah, N.J.: Lawrence Erlbaum Associates. Acknowledges that children do have to learn how to understand the formal features of TV, and discusses how some types of TV filming and editing may affect interpretation.

Hui, L., Boguszewiski, K., & Lillard, A. S. (2015). Can that really happen? Children's knowledge about the reality status of fantastical events in television. *Journal of Experimental Child Psychology*, *139*, 99–114. Although both the studies described here were with older children than my focus here (i.e. 4–6-year-olds), this is still a rare and detailed study of the complexities involved in making reality judgements about moving image media.

Woolley, J. D., & Wellman, H. M. (1990). Young children's understanding of realities, nonrealities and appearances. *Child Development*, *61*, 946–961. Although they do not discuss moving image media, this is a helpful and detailed exploration of the ways in which 1–6-year-olds may develop their thinking about what is and isn't "real."

Discussion

If you have opportunities to watch TV or video with one or more 2–3-year-olds, wait for them to come up with comments about the "reality status" of what they see and hear, and make your own judgments about whether, and how, to encourage further conversation about what they have said. Don't try to initiate a discussion about whether something is "real" or not, unless you have had previous conversations with that child about distinctions between "real" and "pretend."

Reference

Bazalgette, C. (2022). *How toddlers learn the secret language of movies*. Cham, Switzerland: Palgrave Macmillan.

Chapter 9

Learning how to become part of the family culture

Colwyn Trevarthen (1931–2024) was Professor of Child Psychology and Psychobiology at the University of Edinburgh: there's a lot on the internet about him and his work. I found his writing about early childhood quite late in my research and was delighted to find someone who had not only been thinking for a long time on similar lines to mine about how children's capacity for learning develops from birth, but offered me a much deeper understanding about how that learning happens, based on his 25 years of research on babies' development and their relationships with their families. One of the most important features of Trevarthen's work is his inclusion of "culture" in his studies of babies and toddlers:

> Infants can learn, at least from about four months of age, to join in musical or periodic games and dance-like body play...From the interactive rituals of these games with their teasing and jokes comes, by a remarkable internally generated change in the infant's thinking at about nine months after birth, an eagerness to perceive and act *vis a vis* the shared world as others do. The baby, not yet using language, starts to notice trappings of culture, like clothes, books, toys, ways of posing and gesturing, and to use them for 'showing off' the knowledge gained.

The term "culture" tends to get used widely but vaguely by the rest of us, as in "male culture" or "African culture" or "she's a very cultured person," and most of us would be hard put to provide a clear explanation of what it means exactly. For Trevarthen – and also for Tomasello, whom I quote in Chapter 1 – what matters is its communal origin. Trevarthen explains it thus: "Culture ... is an invention of human thoughts, an ordered fantasy for communities that people have agreed to endow with meaning." So unlike common ways of using the word, for example to refer to the characteristics of social groups (as in "working class culture"), or to a set of attitudes (as in "woke culture"), or to artistic works valued by elites (as in "high culture"), Trevarthen and Tomasello use it to include what "everyone" does: almost everyone has family and/or friendship groups – and for some, workplace

DOI: 10.4324/9781003751236-10

groups and maybe leisure activity groups as well – that share similar pleasures, memories, beliefs, activities, possessions, and jokes. The basis of Trevarthen's message is that from birth, babies show their interest in other people and it is this that starts to drive their need to learn (consider my example from Chapter 4 about eye contact with new-borns, and my comment on the seven-week-old Evie in Figure 4.2).

Choosing a TV programme or video to watch is a cultural choice: something we are going to be emotionally affected by, or just enjoy. This is even the case when we make choices for a baby or a toddler, as in "I think she would like this" or "he liked that, so he might like this." And for the child, watching with one or more older children or adults is different from watching it on their own. Even if the co-viewers say nothing, that still communicates a message to the child: "this is interesting" or maybe even "this is funny." Watching with a group is a lot more informative, although it can also be puzzling.

In these kinds of events and dialogues, 0–3s are almost certainly doing two important things: firstly, trying to understand the characters and actions in the stories they are watching; secondly, talking to co-viewers and listening to their comments, while negotiating the meanings they had discovered or worked out for themselves. It doesn't matter if some of their interpretations are wrong. Co-viewing can happen in many ways, depending on the way it works best for each family: it may happen informally, or it may be part of an agreed ritual: after tea and before bedtime, for example. It offers opportunities for pleasurably sharing experiences of family cultures. This is important for small children: not only do they learn more about a programme or film they have already seen, making the story clearer and more meaningful by filling in the gaps; but they also learn more about the roles of TV and film in the family. They may for example overhear comments from older viewers that draw their attention to things they hadn't noticed, or hadn't really understood. There may be references to something or someone that one of the family is reminded of, comparisons to other films or series, guesses about what's going to happen or, if it's a film that everyone has seen before, anticipatory comments such as "I love (or hate) this next bit" and arguments about what might or might not be a misremembering. All of these, whether understood or not, feed into babies' and toddlers' voracious brains. Their learning of "film language" will develop alongside their learning about the culture of their family, and of course their own language learning.

"Learning a culture" is not only something that babies and toddlers do. We all did it when we started school and when we started our first job, and we still do it whenever we enter a new social or professional context or join a leisure activity such as gym exercising or singing in a choir: any new environment that means meeting new people and encountering a new set of procedures, relationships, customs, maybe jokes: all these have their own "cultures" that we like to understand, start sharing in them, and bring in our own contributions. A major part of the pleasure experienced by those of us who enjoy watching *Gogglebox* (Channel 4) is seeing – and then, as we get to know the series, anticipating – the different ways that each couple, family or friendship group responds to the programme they are watching. One couple may exchange dry, cynical remarks; a group of friends may scream with delight or horror; another group of friends may exchange comments about how or why something is happening, or that they anticipate is about to happen. These are all examples of social cultures – though also, of course in this context, examples of showing-off – but they do reflect different, though well-established, patterns of response to shared experiences, reflecting people's knowledge of the genres they like to watch, and the many different patterns of TV audience reactions. If we enjoy anticipating their responses and laughing at some, if not all, of the behaviour we are watching, then that is also part of the "home ground" of our own personal or group culture. And for anyone who would never in a million years want to watch *Gogglebox*: that's also a cultural choice.

We always bring our own past experiences to every new environment that we encounter, which may or may not help us to adjust. In a way, this may also be the case for babies. As I pointed out in Chapter 2, babies do have some pre-birth experiences in the form of the sounds they can hear in the womb: their mother's voice in particular, and more distantly, the voices of others in the family, friends and neighbours, and other sounds such as barking dogs, car engines, and music. So once they are born, they can see the faces that go with some of those voices, feel the hands and arms that grasp and lift them, curl their fingers around a finger offered to them, and hear those more familiar sounds more clearly.

From then on, they never stop learning whenever they are awake. Watching TV and video offers the fascination of seeing different kinds of faces, usually quite unlike the real ones that they see all the time, but nevertheless usually with recognisable eyes and mouths. We all tend to say things like "she loves watching that mobile" or "he always wants to hold that teddy." But we could also think in terms of their drive to learn: she *has* to watch that mobile; he *has* to hold the teddy. One is looking at objects moving in space; the other is feeling texture and shape. And at the same time, both are studying things that are part of their family's culture. It may sound pedantic and odd to refer to these experiences as learning, but if we remember the many times we have each had to adjust to some sort of new environment, we can admit to ourselves that those *were* learning experiences – though nowhere near as huge, significant and potentially daunting as what has to be learned in the first three years of life. Sadly, the word "learning" has accumulated negative connotations on the lines of "it's hard, but we/you have to do it." The research I refer to in Chapter 2, that looks for (and doesn't find) the sort of learning outcomes that the researchers think are important, misses out the extraordinary, self-driven learning that actually is going on – because, of course, most research on children and TV has not used observational techniques in real home environments, and often doesn't recognise the specific characteristics of "film language."

The proliferation of digital devices in the second and third decades of the 21st century is fascinating and useful in many ways, but it does mean for many adults and children that they watch moving image media by themselves. This includes babies and toddlers, who can often be seen in their prams or buggies, gazing at an iPhone in a supermarket or restaurant – where unfortunately they probably can't hear much of the soundtrack of whatever they are watching, but nevertheless may be distracted from whatever they were doing before. I've seen many self-righteous condemnations of this on social media, but it's probably better for the child than having their parent get cross with them.

Parents shouldn't be made to feel self-conscious about what they do and say while watching TV or video with child/ren. Whether or not a child understands any of the comments parents may make, or even if the parents keep quiet while they're watching, the child will still be interested in whatever they do and say while they watch together. This is what's meant by the title of the book that Trevarthen's paper was published in: children *need* to learn the culture of their family, which includes much more than TV, books, pictures, and music. It's about when and why family members talk and when and why they don't, and what they talk about; what they eat and wear; how their rooms are decorated and arranged; their friends and relations (and when – and whether – they see them); the adults' work and how they feel about it; rules like bed time, table manners, and ownership; jokes and stories and much more, including, of course, the stories, jokes, and information that family members get from moving image media, on TV and/or mobile devices, and may share with each other. It's a huge amount of knowledge and understanding that babies have to begin to learn, even when they are still very young, driven by their innate curiosity about everything they can see, hear, and touch.

TAKEAWAYS

Do your own research: Ask friends and/or acquaintances about their family's viewing arrangements when they were young.

Further reading

Trevarthen, C. (1998). The child's need to learn a culture. In M. Woodhead, D. Faulkner, & K. Littleton (Eds.), *Cultural worlds of early childhood*. New York: Routledge.

Student task

Individuals or groups to survey the "culture" of one or more families and present findings to the rest of the group; devise terms to characterise differences.

Chapter 10

Analyses of *Cocomelon* and *Bluey*, and why they're successful

It's easy enough to tell when a toddler – or even a baby – is interested in a video or a TV programme: my comments on the image of Sunu in Chapter 1 point out the indicators of close attention, even at four months. But we can't know what a baby is thinking when she watches TV, or why she wants to go on watching, until her verbal skills have at least reached the stage of one-word exclamations. We can note a baby's attentiveness, and major responses such as fear, but we can't really tell anything much about the extent to which they can follow a story. That hasn't stopped many researchers, TV companies, and parents from making confident assertions about why babies and toddlers like watching moving image media. One claim is that babies, at least, are simply attracted by the colours, movements, and sounds and can't really make any sense of what they are watching. Others (especially the TV companies) argue that programmes of the right sort can offer important early learning opportunities such as counting; probably this is intended to mollify those who still argue that babies and toddlers shouldn't be watching TV at all (in spite of the evidence that most of them are – see "Introduction"), or to challenge those who still believe in the "video deficit effect" (see Chapter 2). Meanwhile, parents' assertions either range from "loves it" to "hypnotised" or "hated it" to "terrified": unless there are notable reactions such as these, parents don't usually have much time to look closely, not even at the child's expressions, let alone at their posture, breathing, and hand positions.

In this chapter, I discuss two examples of TV series for Early Years: the first 30 seconds of a typical 2.51-minute story from the *Cocomelon* series, probably suitable for babies as well as younger toddlers, and the 37-second pre-title sequence of a *Bluey* episode, more suitable for 2.5-year-olds and older. I chose these because of the two very different ways in which they are likely to appeal to viewers in their two different target audiences. I also chose them because they are both series that have been phenomenally successful internationally and are accessible on YouTube, so you may well know one or both of them already. With both, I am providing the kind of very detailed analysis that is more often undertaken only by serious academics analysing "important" feature films. I am doing this here in order to identify

DOI: 10.4324/9781003751236-11

the features of design, script, and editing that older children and adults are able to interpret more or less automatically, but which, on a first viewing, babies and toddlers might find challenging, but maybe also interesting. As I have already argued in earlier chapters, I believe that children will watch a film or video repeatedly if they are intrigued the first time they see it, even if they were puzzled by certain moments, such as a close-up of someone's face followed by a point-of-view shot, or a sudden change of camera angle, emotional expressions being shown when it's not yet clear what the character is reacting to, or, in the quite likely case of *Bluey*, not being able to follow the dialogue. If they feel that there is more to find out, they will probably want to watch it again – maybe many times!

"Old MacDonald song with cute baby farm animals"

Cocomelon developed out of a series of videos on YouTube created by an American, Jay Jeon, which were rebranded as *Cocomelon* in 2018 and are now made by Moonbug Entertainment, which has offices in London and Los Angeles. This stand-alone episode features a toddler, his mother, and their dog, who visit a farm. The toddler encounters the elderly couple who own the farm, and then gets to meet a baby goat, a baby cow, a baby sheep, and some baby chickens (all carefully re-named for him by one of the nearby adults – with subtitles – as kid, calf, lamb, and chicks). The film is made in computer-generated 3D images (CGI) animation and the 30-second section I'm going to discuss has 10 shots. That's an average of three seconds per shot, so although the textures, shapes, and colours of the film are very smooth and gentle, the pace is brisk. The visual style uses several traditional cinematic devices: point-of-view shots, high and low camera angles, etc. (see Chapter 3). The action all seems to take place in one continuous time-sequence. I will use terms such as "camera angle" and "shots" in my analysis, although of course the film was actually constructed with computer animation software. It is easy to find this episode online at www.youtube.com/watch?v=cp9IucnYj_Q (accessed March 2026).

The shot that starts the film is a low-angle view of Mom, Kid, and Dog walking "towards us" along a country road (the characters' nicknames are invented by me: the film doesn't name them). Kid is laughing and we can hear cheerful music, starting with a xylophone playing the introductory phrase of the song "Old MacDonald had a Farm." Behind them is the reverse side of the type of wooden sign that might be familiar to US children, and to those British viewers who have seen Westerns: it's the traditional-style gateway to a farm or a ranch. The whole film is full of "traditional" images of farming.

After three seconds, there is a cut to a reverse shot (i.e. to show what and who the two are walking towards, from their point of view). At the same low angle but from behind Kid, who is walking forwards with outstretched arms, we can see ahead of him a plump, white-moustached man in dungarees and check shirt, and a grey-haired woman in a skirt and cardigan, both standing about four metres away and waving excitedly (adults will know that they must be "the farmer and his wife"). Behind them, there's a wooden gate and fence, and behind those are buildings and trees. As Kid starts to walk towards the farmers, there's a short burst of drum beats, with a flute starting to play the Old Macdonald melody.

Two seconds later there is a jump-cut (i.e. the film's story-time leaves out a few seconds of action) to a low-angle reverse shot, which shows Kid now already walking towards us excitedly between Wife and Farmer as they open the double sides of the gate and all three walk through. It is framed so that we can just see one leg and one hand of each adult and Kid from his hips upwards: we can recognise Farmer and Wife by their clothes. Farmer's hand swings, wrist upwards, and palm forward, in a "welcome" gesture. The Kid is laughing, and as he comes closer his face almost fills the screen, with eyebrows raised and his huge eyes opening even wider as he stops for a moment and gasps. We can see from this shot that he is supposed to be around 12–18 months old, as he just has two top incisor teeth – so probably the same age as the main target audience. He is wearing a sleeveless top (or perhaps a bib) over his check shirt, which has a picture of a pony on it, with a baby chick jumping off its back, and some musical notes decorate the background.

As we hear Kid exclaim "Wow!" there is a cut to a very high-angle view of the whole farmyard with the four characters still in the same positions as in the previous shot, but from this vantage point looking very tiny. This sets the scene for the encounters that Kid is about to have. The shot includes a detail that would probably take more than two seconds to notice, but which might be recognised during re-viewings: a few metres away from Kid is the tiny white-dot figure of the baby goat he is about to meet. But this sudden cutaway to a long-distance view, though very brief, is quite strange in narrative terms, given that it follows immediately after Kid exclaiming "wow!" but it certainly doesn't show us his point of view. So it could be intriguing, or it might be confusing, at least on first viewing, especially for inexperienced viewers – but it is very short.

Back at ground level two seconds later, Kid moves forward, out of the shot, leaving the Farmers standing on each side of the gate, with Mother and Dog still approaching. We hear a child's voice joining the music, singing the song "Old MacDonald had a farm" with an adult male voice joining in the "E-I-E-I-O" chorus. The words are subtitled in green lettering that changes to red as the song progresses (either to support anyone who wants to try and read it or, for younger children, just to be aware that the letters they see relate to the words they hear). There is a cut to Shot 6: a close-up to show the wooden gates swinging shut, with Mom and Dog still outside: Dog peers through the gate and blinks, as the next line of the song plays "And on his farm was a baby goat." A cut to Shot 7 shows Kid trotting towards the brown-and-white baby goat, which closes its eyes blissfully and dances from one foot to another as Kid approaches. As the word "goat" is sung, there is a cut to Shot 8: a close-up of the baby goat, who is being patted by someone's hand. A cut to Shot 9 shows us whose hand it is: Farmer, kneeling on one knee, is patting the baby goat's head and then straightens up to look directly at us, saying "a baby goat is called a kid," spreading both hands as he does so. Immediately there is a cut to Shot 10: a mid-shot of Kid jumping excitedly, spreading his arms and shouting "yeah!" as the goat kid runs behind him and the chorus "with a meh-meh here, and a meh-meh there" begins.

This is quite a lot of information for a 30-second sequence. In ten shots we are introduced to six characters, their relationships, an animal, and a large setting. I find it interesting that the editing style makes few concessions for a toddler audience, unless one includes the emphasis in the script and the emphasis on learning the correct words for the baby animals (perhaps a reaction to those researchers who believe in the "Video Deficit Effect" and claim that children learn nothing from TV-watching – see Chapter 2). There is no voice-over telling the viewer who these characters are, and the editing follows the long-established conventions of cinema, with changes of angle, switches from one point of view to another, and extremely fast cutting: many of the shots last only two seconds. There is no dialogue: character, relationships, and emotions are all conveyed by facial expressions, body language, and music. However, the major "toddler-friendly" features are the simplified features, big eyes (for the animals as well as the humans), and enormous heads – especially Kid's. It is his eyes, eyebrows, and mouth that convey his reactions – always delighted, amazed, or blissfully content. So the immediate and major "messages" of the film are emotional: excitement, anticipation, friendliness, affection, and surprise. The rest of the film introduces the other baby animals one by one and ends up with the dog surprising everyone by hiding inside a pile of straw and bursting out of the top of it, supposedly looking like a "baby lion" because lots of straw stalks have got stuck to its collar, slightly like a lion's mane.

These stylistic and design features would obviously reward re-viewing. Fast cutting and frequent changes of viewpoint may well not be clear to a toddler the first time she sees them, but they are likely to make more sense each time she watches the film. It is this that has alarmed many critics: the producers' research on what kind of visual style would appeal to babies and toddlers identified this as one that would hold their attention: it is this that Jessica Sannes and other critics have seized on as "sinister," although to me it is *Cocomelon*'s one redeeming feature amidst the otherwise relentless cheeriness. The simplified shapes and smooth textures are very bland, but the emphasis on facial expressions and the different states of mind that they convey are clearly meant to appeal to babies as well as to toddlers. The worlds that the *Cocomelo*n films convey are designed to be reassuring, to promote kindliness and pleasure – and on the way, to establish that a baby sheep is a LAMB.

"No more squabbles!"

Bluey is another, very different TV series for toddlers and pre-schoolers, created by Joe Brumm, an Australian animator, director, and writer who worked on a number of British TV series including *Peppa Pig*, before returning to Australia to start his own company. He planned a TV series inspired by his experience on *Peppa Pig*, which became *Bluey*, the hugely successful series made by a Queensland studio, Ludo. It was originally commissioned by the Australian Broadcasting Commission in partnership with the BBC, launched in 2018 and by 2026 was broadcast in over 50 countries. At the time of writing this book, over 150 episodes had been made and a feature film was being planned for 2027, in partnership with Disney. *Bluey* has won many awards, and is even commended in *Psychology Today* as a "masterclass in parenting" (Routledge, 2025). One example of the huge amount of enthusiasm that *Bluey* has generated can be seen in an excited article by "Dr Elizabeth" in www.parents.com (Elizabeth, 2025), describing research by academics at Central Queensland University that counted the number of "resilience messages" in all 150 episodes of *Bluey,* concluding that the series is "a strong example of how children's television can support emotional learning and model adaptive behaviours relevant to real-life challenges" (Bohl et al., 2024). I am guessing that the relaxation of the AAP's "screen time" rule and the emergence of radical new series such as *Bluey* has begun to open up a wider range of research opportunities for academics who are as tired as I am of the well-worn "TV is bad for kids" mantra, and also ready – at last – to acknowledge the role of "good parenting" in children's lives, although for many parents this may also be worrying and guilt-inducing.

For those few readers who have never seen *Bluey*: you need to know that it is focused on a family of Australian "heelers" ("a popular breed of dog that are known for their intelligence, loyalty, and strong work ethic," according to www.vetexplainspets.com), otherwise known as "cattle dogs." Some heelers do have blue-grey fur that is characterised as "blue." The series characters consist of Dad ("Bandit"), Mum ("Chilli"), and two daughters: "Bingo," aged four, and "Bluey," aged six. The visual style of *Bluey* is very different from *Cocomelon:* the characters have highly simplified outlines and are quite flat-looking, with fur indicated only by spiky outlines. Although depth of field is indicated by the perspectival features of furniture, walls, etc., and when the characters (who are all dogs) turn sideways or – as they do in the title sequence – dance, turn around, or run away, we do see other features of their bodies: their arms and their tails. Each character has a faint oval patch of "shadow" under them, but otherwise there are no indications of three dimensions, except in the perspectival adjustments when characters or vehicles move towards or away from us. The colours are all soft pastel shades and the indoor scenes are basic in design: there's just enough detail to indicate which sort of room we're in (living room, study, kitchen, bedroom). Exteriors can be more elaborate: for example, episodes that involve a trip to the "creek" show rich foliage and flowers, and others involving a trip to the beach show a huge panorama of sand and ocean waves. Otherwise, we are in a quiet suburban neighbourhood.

The characters' appearance is only dog-like in that they have big pricked-up ears, tails, and hind paws (functioning as feet). Their fat little hands are the classic three-fingered cartoon hands (so not like dogs OR humans). Despite all this simplification, their huge oval eyes, sausage-like eyebrows that can move independently of their faces, and their highly mobile mouths, all serve to express emotions such as excitement, friendliness, surprise, annoyance, guilt, anxiety, pleading, and so on. These are a vital part of the series' project: every episode involves the negotiation of relationships, behaviour, and desires. The characters don't wear clothes – which may have allowed many new viewers (including me) to assume on their first viewing that Bluey is male. They all have the same pattern of body markings, with darker colours on their heads and lighter colours on their snouts, bellies, hands, feet, and tail tips (so, very slightly like real Heelers) and are distinguished from one another mainly by size and colour: Bandit and Bluey are both blue with brown snouts, hands, feet, and bellies; Chilli and Bingo are brown, with off-white snouts, hands, feet, and bellies. The only really dog-like thing is that they all have shiny black noses. Their eyes, eyebrows, mouths, and hands constantly express emotions, but only as an accompaniment to the dialogue, which can claim to be the most significant part of the series. The adults are voiced by adults, and the children by children, all with Australian accents.

The combination of simple graphics and quick-fire dialogue is well-illustrated in the 38-second first part of the Highlight (i.e. "short") episode called "Postman" (Bluey Season 2, available at www.youtube.com/watch?v=9JZc7s_GVPI). It opens with Bluey, centre screen, eating something from a plate on the coffee table and Bingo coming into the living-room from Screen Left. There is a brief dialogue between them, in which Bingo asks to play a game called "Ground is Lava" and Bluey agrees, pointing out that you can't touch the ground in that game. Bingo jumps excitedly, yelling "yeah" and Bluey says "OK! I'll just take my plate back to the kitchen" walking towards Screen Right, carrying her plate. There's a cut back to Bingo, jumping on to the coffee table with an excited giggle. Then there's a cut to Chilli and Bandit, standing facing each other in the kitchen, in what turns out to be the middle of an argument:

[MID-SHOT] **Chilli:** "I see what you're saying, I just don't agree!"
Bandit*:* (crossly) "How can you not agree?"

[WIDE-SHOT] **Bluey** (entering, Screen Right, carrying a plate) "Are you two quarrelling?"
Chilli*:* (gesturing) "One second, Bluey"
[MID-SHOT] **Bandit:** (still looking at Chilli, gesturing, and then folding his arms) "If you attach the bin to the door, it means I have to touch the bin bags!"
Chilli: (loudly, and slamming the under-sink cupboard door)" Yeah! But you *don't have* to touch the bin!"
[WIDE SHOT] **Bandit:** "*But I like taking the whole bin out*! Bin bags are a pain!" (folding arms).
Bluey, holding her plate, starts to run forward from the side of the screen.
Chilli: (rolling her eyes and then half-lowering her eyelids) "**You're** a pain!"
[MID-SHOT] **Bandit:** "oh, great" (then he sees Bluey, coming to a halt between them and stretching her arms out to both parents)
[CLOSE-UP] **Bluey:** (crossly) "Stop squabbling, I don't like it!" (Both parents look down at her, surprised).
Bandit: "We're not squabbling, kiddo, we're just talking!
Chilli: (bending forward) "Sorry, Bluey, it's OK.
[MID-SHOT] **Chilli:** (to Bandit, while walking forwards and then out of shot, Screen Left)
"Look, let's talk about it later"
Bandit: (with ironically half-lowered eyelids) "Can't wait!"

CUT TO TITLE ON PLAIN BLUE BACKGROUND: "POSTMAN"
VO: (child's voice) "This episode of *Bluey* is called "Postman."
The remaining 1.31 minutes of the episode are taken up with Bluey organising her parents into writing letters to each other, in order to make up for what Bandit persists in calling "a discussion." Chilli is still in the house; Bandit is outside hammering nails into what may be a broken bit of fence. Bluey claims that their exchange in the kitchen was a squabble, to which Bandit replies "maybe, but we still love each other" as he writes his letter, folds it up, and gives it to Bluey. In her "postman" role as she goes back to the house, Bluey sneaks a look at the "letter," which turns out to be a big drawing of a red heart, with "I" above it and "U" below, signed off from "DAD." Then she goes back to Bingo and starts the "ground is lava" game at last. A sequel to this episode, called "The Floor is Lava" shows Bluey and Bingo nearly having a quarrel when Bluey is on her way to "post" the letter and Bingo accuses her of always making promises and not keeping them. But they then agree that it was only an argument and that they can go ahead and play what is called "The Floor is Lava!" when they are in the house and can use household equipment to ride on and not "burn their feet" in the imaginary lava.

With just over 5 seconds per shot, this episode of *Bluey* is slightly less tightly cut than the *Cocomelon* episode that I described earlier, but substantially different in its fast dialogue. As the show started after I had finished my PhD research, I haven't observed babies or toddlers viewing any of the episodes. Given that dialogue is important in every episode, I believe that the online comments suggesting that is it appropriate for ages two to seven are plausible, though I doubt that many toddlers younger than two and a half (apart from Australian ones) can follow the fast-talking Australian-accented voices that dominate the action, and maybe not always understand how the arguments are resolved. Bandit and Chilli are easier to understand, with their louder and slower speech, and there are many opportunities for older viewers to enjoy the silly arguments that precede each good-humoured reconciliation. The clothing and toy merchandising that relate to the show range from babies to much older children, and many adults love *Bluey*, judging by online comments and social media threads, so presumably a lot of older children enjoy it too. So do I!

The puppies Bluey and Bingo are central to every *Bluey* episode. Although they have "puppy" faces, ears, and tails, they walk on two legs and children can easily identify with them, as well as their numerous puppy friends. The parents, Bandit and Chilli, also play a key role in most of the narratives. Child viewers are likely to enjoy the resourceful, sensible, and adventurous puppy characters, while adults can be wryly amused by the interactions between puppies and parents, in which the adults are not only sources of wisdom and practicality but can also be caught out making misjudgements or (as in the Postman episode) having to apologise. And anyone who still grimly adheres to the belief that TV cannot possibly be of any benefit to children should be made to sit down and watch the Sleepytime episode (Series 2, episode 26).

When I looked in March 2026, there were 431 journal articles related to *Bluey* listed in my university's library. I confess that I didn't read them all, but from those that I did, I could see two recurrent themes in the literature. Internationally, and predictably, the series has been seized upon as (at last?) a children's TV series which is not only impossible to attack as a sinister threat to toddlers' later development, but can even be praised for promoting resilience (see earlier references), for exemplifying "good parenting" (Rutledge, 2025) and as being a series that appeals to a wide age-range. One article explores the new phenomenon of a "distributed fandom affinity space," as a way of characterising the hundreds of parents who tweet under the hashtag #Bluey (Dynel & Ross, 2022).

But also, from a specifically Australian point of view, there is excitement about the way *Bluey* represents and celebrates Australian culture and landscapes, for example:

> *Bluey* follows the daily lives of a family of anthropomorphised Australian Cattle Dogs: a 6-year-old blue heeler Bluey, her younger sister Bingo and their parents Bandit and Chilli. The show is set in semi-tropical North Queensland and is stocked with signifiers of everyday Australian life, including native wildlife, backyard BBQs and "verandah Santas."
>
> (Balanzategui et al., 2020)

Thus, *Bluey* has opened up a space for developing arguments about the wider cultural value of animations for children, including the possibility of showing and discussing them in educational contexts. For example, a study by Arigata-Garcia and others describes their analysis of the 52 episodes in the first season of *Bluey*, identifying 3327 cultural and societal facets of Australian culture that those episodes depicted, and arguing that such a compilation would facilitate "a nuanced approach to teaching English, rooted in the diverse and culturally rich Australian context, thus breaking away from strictly British and American cultural associations and embracing a broader linguistic and cultural landscape" (Arigata-Garcia et al., 2024). They saw *Bluey* as "an invaluable resource for enriching the cultural learning of the English language and culture from an Australian point of view, an issue that is rarely addressed in the specialist literature." I don't think it is too much of a stretch to consider *Bluey* – or maybe other series that may eventually follow in its wake – as similar resources for supporting those toddlers in UK Early Years settings who are adapting to a new language and culture.

There are therefore enormous differences in style between these two very successful series: *Cocomelon* and *Bluey*. The *Cocomelon* film employs "classical" film editing conventions from the very start (shot/reverse shot, point-of-view shots, etc.) in an extremely rapid series, while its overall "look" has the clean lines, simplified figures, soft colours and huge heads that are typical of many CGI series. The toddler main character is shown repeatedly in very large close-ups which display his emotions though his huge eyes, eyebrows and mouth, and his gasps and laughs. Bluey is much funnier, and offers pleasures to a much wider range of viewers. Both series have earned vast amounts of revenue through international sales and also through advertising. Both also receive income through licensed sales of toys and books.

Cocomelon's rapid pace, combined with the frequent close-ups of Kid's excited reactions, may accustom a child to shot changes that reflect instinctive behaviour in real life, such as point-of-view shots: the point where Kid looks suddenly toward the right side of the screen, with wide eyes and a gasp, which is followed by a cut to an image of the calf, is a clear example, though there are many in the film, given that it is all about the exploration of the farmyard environment. Another cut from shot to shot – the switch at 14 seconds to a very high point of view of the whole farm yard – is not clearly motivated, in that it is not a point of view held by any of the characters. But although the pace of the film is so fast, young viewers won't be puzzled for long: the narrative is extremely simple, and constantly reverts to close-ups of Kid's face to show his reactions, which are always excited and pleased, so episodes are likely to be understood easily: if not on a first viewing. Research by the *Cocomelo*n producers apparently found that this relatively sophisticated style would attract and retain very young viewers: this is what many critics have deemed "addictive" – in other words, sinister. Obviously, I don't think it is sinister at all: it's just a recognition of what babies and toddlers are doing when they watch moving image material that they like.

There are, then, major differences between the "projects" of these two series. *Bluey*'s style is in one sense much less visually realistic than *Cocomelon*'s, but emotionally it is more "true to life." There are no highlights to show the roundedness of bodies, or shading to indicate bodily shapes, and no indication of the textures of bodies, furniture, or objects. We are rarely offered point-of-view shots: characters perform as if on a stage, with little indication of depth of field. It is the dialogue, both as text and in performance, which is very realistic. Although the Australian accents may be a little difficult for some Anglophone speakers in other countries, viewers get used to these quite easily, especially when they can have repeated viewings. And the inclusion of Holst's "Planets" suite in the "Sleepytime" episode (Season 2m, no 26) is a triumphant innovation for baby-and-toddler TV.

Cocomelon presents souped-up versions of places, relationships, and behaviour that obviously claim to represent real life, despite the fact that everything is shown in the exaggerated *Cocomelon* style: enormous heads, hugely expressive eyes, frequent cuts to close-ups, and to point-of-view shots. The style of the series emphasises colour and texture. The appeal is to quite a narrow range of emotions, and the project is to emphasise good behaviour: kindness and friendliness, but without any references to unkind or unfriendly behaviour. The *Bluey* characters don't look at all like us, but this is counteracted by the highly believable voices and familiar-sounding dialogue: there can be disagreements, but they always get resolved, and often are discussed as well, but not loaded with reaction shots, as happens in many *Cocomelon* episodes. A significant difference between the two series is that there are almost no conflicts or problems in *Cocomelon*, but many in *Bluey*. *Cocomelon* can therefore feel bland, whereas Bluey not only shows disagreements and disappointments, but presents emotionally realistic accounts of how they can be resolved.

TAKEAWAYS

View one or more TV programmes or YouTube offerings that are aimed at the 0–3 age range, preferably one that is watched in families that you are in contact with. Use "baby and toddler TV" as a search term if you are looking online. Try your own analysis of one instalment or even just one scene – refer back to Chapter 3 if you need to recall types of shots and transitions. Consider what might be challenging for a very young viewer.

Choose one or more of the references to follow up and read in detail. Write your own review of an episode from either series, providing your own opinion on their suitability for children in the 2–3 age range.

References

Arigata-Garcia, A., Mañoso-Pacheco, L.,, Estrada-Chichon J. L., & Snachez-Cabraro R. (2024). Mapping Australian culture and society in the animated series bluey—The use of audiovisual material in early EFL learning. *Societies, 14*(252). https://doi.org/10.3390/soc14120252

Balanzategui, J., Burke, L., & McIntyre J. (2020). 'What would Bandit do?': Reaffirming the educational role of Australian children's television during the COVID-19 pandemic and beyond. *Media International Australia, 178*(1).

Bohl, K. A., Smith, Bradley P., Bolling, Mary T. (2024). "Oh, Biscuits!" Exploring resilience in the children's television programme *Bluey. Educational and Developmental Psychologist, 42*(2).

Dynel, M., & Ross, A. S. (2022). Metarecipient parents' #Bluey tweets as a distributed fandom affinity space. *Poetics (Amsterdam), 92*. https://doi.org/10.1016/j.poetic.2022.101648

Elizabeth, D. (2025, September 10, 2022). [Parents]. Retrieved from www.parents.com/researchers-analyzed-150-episodes-of-bluey-to-find-its-most-powerful-theme-11807168

Rutledge, P. B. (2025). 7 reasons why "Bluey" is a masterclass in parenting. *Psychology Today*. Retrieved from www.psychologytoday.com/us/blog/positively-media/202503/7-reasons-why-bluey-is-a-masterclass-in-parenting

Chapter 11

How viewing skills develop: "using it up" and "moving on"

However much a toddler enjoys a TV series or a short film, there will come a time when he has "used it up," by which I mean that he has extracted all the meaning and pleasure it had to offer, and is ready for something else. If he has one or more older siblings, they may well be watching material that he doesn't understand, but that he may watch anyway, especially if they take moments to explain things to him. Or he may just drift away and do something else. His siblings or parents may come across something they think he'll want to watch, perhaps by searching online or chatting to other parents. Before long, he'll move on to a new programme or series that interests him.

I was a bit taken aback when the twins, then aged 2 years 7 months, started to watch *Tree Fu Tom,* four months after its release on CBeebies (it ran until 2016 and is still available on BBC iPlayer). They had been watching toddler series such as *Peppa Pig* and *Numtums*; *Tree Fu Tom* is considerably different from them. Although it is mainly animated and the running time of each episode is approximately the same as *Peppa Pig*, it includes animated action sequences with extremely fast cutting between shots, and some excited direct address to viewers by the characters themselves, to which the viewers are supposed to respond. But the most significant differences between it and what the twins had been watching were its complexity, numerous very odd characters (each based on a different woodland creature), high-speed narration, and a different problem to solve in each episode. I wondered whether they'd really understand it enough to enjoy it. I was wrong – the twins loved it, enjoyed quoting from it, and imitating the characters. I have described the series and their relationship with it in more detail in my earlier book (Bazalgette, 2022).

Based on a classic trope of fantasy drama, exploited by many toy manufacturers, that donning a certain garment or accessory will transform you into someone with magical powers, the basis of all the *Tree Fu Tom* stories is that Tom, an ordinary boy who lives in a cottage beside a wood, has a magic belt that, once he straps it on, enables him to become a miniature superhero as he flies up into the hidden world of Treetopolis, which is entered via a tree close to his home. That is the live-action sequence that starts every episode: as

DOI: 10.4324/9781003751236-12

Tom zooms up into the tree, he becomes a tiny animated figure. The whole Treetopolis world is CGI-animated as well. Every episode moves at a frenetic pace, with fast cutting and numerous changes of angle, so rewards repeat viewing.

In Treetopolis, Tom has adventures with many characters, all versions of woodland creatures and plants such as an acorn, a tree frog, a butterfly, a woodlouse, and a spider, which all move and talk at an excited, loud, quick-fire pace. The characters are more complex and more differentiated than the fantasy figures in most toddler TV series. Some have jobs; these include, for example, ranch manager, inventor, and "sap miner." All have different backgrounds, abilities, and specialisms. There is also an overall "wise woman" character called Treetog the Tree Spirit, who oversees Treetopolis and teaches magic. A feature that is significantly different from most things the twins had watched before was the presence of two unpleasant characters: the toadstools Puffy and Stink, whose machinations form the plot device in some episodes, and have to be overcome by Tom and his friends: Twigs (an "acorn sprite") and Ariel (an American-accented butterfly, who looks after the "Branch Ranch" which is populated by numerous insects). The fact that Puffy and Stink are both fat, look different from all the other characters (not that those look all the same either) and don't generate any sympathy, might raise concerns about representations of diversity.

However, *Tree Fu Tom* certainly presents viewers with a lot to remember, considerably more narrative complexity than in most baby and toddler TV, and the new concept that there can be bad people, who commit actions that have to be countered and remedied. The Treetopolis community has its own rules and customs and the characters are very distinct from one another. Unlike *Peppa Pig*, there is no narrator commenting on the events and plot developments: viewers have to work these out for themselves, always depending in part on the characters' different interests and specialisms, and helped by their tendency to shout frequent explanations to each other.

A feature of *Tree Fu Tom* which distinguishes its relationship with audiences is that it was developed in association with the Dyspraxia Foundation, to encourage children with developmental coordination disorder to perform specific exercises. So each episode includes scenes at key moments of danger, when Tom suddenly faces the camera, addressing the audience directly and asking for help by demonstrating a series of movements that he says will generate the large quantities of "big world magic" that are needed to solve the current problem – but there will only be enough if all the children watching can immediately do them too. Despite the likelihood that many (if not most) children watching the show won't bother to get up and do these exercises, the "big world magic" (represented by a stream of glittery stuff) quickly flows back into the scene anyway from the sides and corners of the screen. The problem – for example, characters in the story being attacked by "sticky bugs" – is always immediately resolved and Tom thanks the audience for their "help."

The twins found these interludes silly and boring, although Alfie did enjoy (somewhat ironically) imitating the call for "big world magic" to make something happen which he knew was about to happen anyway: opening tube train doors, for example. Connie was less impressed by this feature of the series and just waited for each one – which only lasted about a minute – to end. Neither of them ever tried doing the exercises. The series' attraction for them seemed to lie in the diversity and weirdness of the characters and the frenetic pace of each 24-minute episode. Connie also particularly liked Ariela who, with her glamorous appearance, wide practical knowledge, terrific strength, reliable fearlessness, and American accent, was a much more exciting role model than Peppa Pig.

My children (Ben and Phoebe) were aged 27 and 25, respectively, had already left home and were living in different countries when the animated 92-minute feature film *Monsters, Inc.* (USA 2021) was released in the UK in February 2002, so they had no personal experience of enjoying it as young children. Nevertheless, they both introduced their own two-year-old children to it. Ben, living in Italy, quickly acquired a video of the film which he and his partner and their son Morgan (born in 2001) watched together – Morgan's own, self-driven replay of a funny but also potentially frightening scene, when he was 27 months old, is described in Chapter 7.

The twins were initially indifferent to the complex concepts that the film is based on, its wisecracking dialogue and satirical portrayal of corporate culture. Nevertheless, after they had acquired the toy version of the one-eyed, blob-shaped central character Mike Wazowski, and seen the film once or twice more, they became devoted to it and were greatly distressed each time it approached its inevitable end. Like Morgan at a similar age, they were then just about able to watch a full-length feature, and demanded several re-viewings.

Parents are best-placed to judge whether their child may be ready to watch a feature film, although it can well happen that a child with older siblings may get to see bits, if not all, of a film they are watching. It is unlikely that a toddler less than three years old will be able to follow a complete feature film on first viewing. If it doesn't make sense to them, they'll probably soon give up, but they may try to understand it, and may well enjoy watching it anyway if it is spectacular and/or beautiful, especially if older family members are watching it too.

Parents may find it alarming, or at least boring, if their child/ren want to watch a feature film several times., but it is understandable that it is quite a challenge for a three-year-old to assemble all the information they need to understand a film of 90 minutes or more. One way that feature film-viewing may be introduced to a toddler is when older siblings and/or parents may be keen to re-view something they are fond of and hope that the smaller child/ren will be able to watch it too (see also my discussion of "social viewing" in Chapter 9).

It can work very well if parents can find a feature film that they recall with pleasure and that has a relatively simple plot. My husband Terry Staples had run the National Film Theatre's junior screenings for many years, and had had many successes with older, general-audience films that were enjoyed by family audiences, which sometimes included toddlers. He, Phoebe, and I all had fond memories of the musical *Mary Poppins* (Disney 1964) which we'd taken Phoebe and her brother to see when they were respectively about six and eight years old, but we tried it out on the twins when they were 29 months old.

We began by just playing some of the song and dance numbers. The twins were fascinated. A scene that we loved – for its wild dancing and total disregard for workplace safety compliance – was the 3.45-minute Step in Time sequence (available on YouTube) in which the music gets faster and faster as the chimney sweeps dance and leap around on the rooftops in the dark as they sing, embarking on ever more risky movements, including jumping over to the neighbouring house and back again, and one dancer swinging another out over the four-storey drop to the street. Mary Poppins, and the two children to whom she is nursemaid, sit on a chimney stack, watching this delightedly, and as soon as the sweeps' dance ends at 2.5 minutes; Mary gets up to dance with Bert, shaking her red skirts and at one point revealing her ability to take off into the air, much to the sweeps' surprise. Alfie stood close to the screen (this was at their house, where the TV was on a higher shelf) and watched the whole sequence intently – I could see his head following the swirling movements of Mary's dress as she wove in and out of the chorus of sweeps. In contrast, Connie sat on Phoebe's lap, straight-faced and anxious, as we three adults chortled at the way the scene combines ridiculous excessiveness with terrific dancing skills.

Another success was *The Wizard of Oz* (USA 1939). There were, however, several failures. She tried *Bugsy Malone* (USA/UK 1976), but the twins were terrified by the splurge guns and refused to watch it again. She had high hopes of *The Princess Bride* (USA 1976), but it was too sophisticated and the torture scene was too much for them, being much too realistic by comparison with the Randall torture scene in *Monsters, Inc.* (see also Chapter 7). Her biggest failure was with *Dumbo* (USA 1941): once Dumbo's mother was shut in a cage, all three of them burst into tears and for her own sake she was never able to try showing it to them again.

Hannah Wojciechowski, an American literary theorist, has a theory about what goes on in our brains when we watch films. She uses an account of consciousness by a French neuroscientist, Dehaene, who argues that no one can really hold two thoughts in their mind at the same time, even though we like to think that we can. Based on this, Wojciechowski chooses "diakrisis" (a Greek word meaning "discernment") to refer to the ways in which experienced viewers can, constantly and almost automatically, pick out and remember the most salient bits of the mass of information that a film is throwing at them all the time (Wojciechowski, 2015). We can select, and recall, even quite fleeting images or little bits of dialogue, which we identify as being significant to the development of the story. This is obviously a skill that younger children have to take time to develop, so musicals can be an enjoyable "way in" to longer films, given the way that song and dance sequences can help to consolidate the emotional dimensions of a story.

Most of the feature films and the more complex TV series that child viewers are likely to move on to in their third year make increasing demands on children's linguistic abilities, as well as on their memories. So re-viewing them, perhaps more than once – and talking about them afterwards – can enhance children's fluency and vocabulary, as well as stimulating their imagination. That's not to argue that children *ought* to be watching feature films. Family circumstances and preferences will obviously affect what kinds of viewing experiences children have access to. For some, the decision to take a child on a first-time visit to a cinema to see a feature film may be seen as a special treat, which can be an amazing experience for a small child. I well remember taking Phoebe (aged 4) to see *The Wizard of Oz* in a cinema: at the end she refused to move from her seat, but sat there angrily kicking the seat in front of her and growling "I WANT MORE!" (a desire that was satisfied many times over in the subsequent 46 years). Some children may find the cinema experience overwhelming and beg to be taken out, but my experiences of many attendances at children's cinema club screenings indicates to me that it's quite rare for that to happen. It may be necessary to whisper explanations to a child, so a good children's cinema club manager should announce that parents are free to do this and the rest of the audience should not object.

Seeing feature films on video or online to start with does at least allow for pauses to explain things, for stopping altogether if it turns out to be not a good choice of film, for time to chat about it afterwards, either straight away or later on, and of course the opportunity to watch it again soon. It can be quite challenging for some children to deal with the change from watching a series, where the episodes are unlikely to be more than 30 minutes at most –often much shorter – and viewers have time to get used to characters and conventions, to following a feature film of 90 minutes or more. Watching a film at home does allow for pauses and repetitions if they seem necessary. Having opportunities to watch full-length feature films from time to time can be a valuable extension of a three-year-old's interpretive skills in making sense of moving image media, and films from a different era or a genre that is new to them can introduce them to styles and conventions that are intriguingly different. In the case of new films that the parents themselves haven't seen, they will probably want to preview the film if they can, or at least check out the trailer online, and look for reviews. It may be a safe option is for parents to show their children a film that they themselves enjoyed as a child and, of course, to watch it with them.

TAKEAWAYS

Recall a feature film that you saw when you were young: write about, or discuss with others, what you can recall and how it affected you.

Further reading

Staples, T. (1997). *All pals together: The story of children's cinema*. Edinburgh University Press.

References

Bazalgette, C. (2022). *How toddlers learn the secret language of movies*. Cham, Switzerland: Palgrave Macmillan.

Wojciechowski, H. C. (2015). The floating world: Film narrative and viewer diakresis. In M. Coegnarts & P. Kravanja (Eds.), *Embodied cognition and cinema*. Leuven: Leuven University Press.

Chapter 12

Institutional and policy contexts of baby-and-toddler TV and video

Despite the research evidence that 75% of UK babies watch TV (see "Introduction"), the Early Years frameworks and curricula in all four UK nations make no mention of how practitioners might engage with that activity. Of course, this is not very surprising. Despite the AAP's modification of the "screen time" rules from 2016 onwards and the UK's milder new guidance in 2026, negative opinions of TV and VOD continue to circulate and persist, such as: they are irrelevant, if not actually hazardous, to infant and toddler development, who can only watch "passively," and that parents who allow them to watch are being irresponsible. An explicit inclusion of references to TV or video in the Early Years frameworks could generate a storm of press outrage. But this is very unlikely, given that the only British agency that could take on responsibility for developing official advice about what audiences need to understand about media now has to be Ofcom, the British Office of Communications, established by the Department for Culture, Media and Sport (DCMS) in 2002 as a public corporation, accountable to Parliament as the regulator and competition authority for the UK's communication industries, but also with "a duty to promote media literacy."

Adding media literacy to Ofcom's remit might be seen as an odd decision. It arrived through political contexts and processes that are described and analysed by Buckingham and Wallis in their 2013 article for the *European Journal of Communication* (Wallis & Buckingham, 2013) In a second article, for the *International Journal of Public Policy* in 2016, they explain how the decision to give responsibility to a regulatory body for what would normally be a concern for educators meant that "media literacy's broader educative purposes, so clearly articulated in much of the early policy rhetoric, [are] effectively marginalized" (Wallis & Buckingham, 2016). By "early policy rhetoric" they mean, for example, the journal *Screen Education* in the 1970s, the efforts undertaken by the British Film Institute's Education Department (which is where I worked) from the 1980s onwards, and over the same period by the then independent Institute of Education (now part of University College London). Ofcom's remit has included "media literacy" since it was first established, although this term was not widely used in the

DOI: 10.4324/9781003751236-13

UK in 2002. The New Labour administration selected the term from the USA, and ignored the fact that it was "media education" that was then starting to find a toehold in the education provision of all four UK nations, although the DCMS was well aware of this, since funding the BFI was, and is, one of their responsibilities.

The DCMS also ignored a 1999 report entitled *Making Movies Matter,* about the importance and potential of education about film. They themselves had commissioned it from a "Film Education Working Group" that they had set up, which consisted of 25 people representing a wide range of experience: some in teaching and writing about film, others in film making, distribution or training, which convened at the BFI. It is possible that the DCMS backtracked on the idea of promoting either "film education" or "media education" when they realised that demanding the development of either would place new and unknown pressures on an education system that was already overwhelmed with other demands, and that they saw "media literacy,"," despite its vagueness, as a better way of signalling that they would be encouraging audiences to be selective and critical about what they watched on screens of any kind. They would also not have wanted to interfere in anything that would have been the responsibility of the Department of Education. These factors may have made them decide that it would be appropriate to add it to Ofcom's remit, and to let them figure out what it meant and how to make it happen. As Wallis and Buckingham argue, choosing the term "media literacy" and awarding responsibility for it to Ofcom without any supporting definition weakened the chances of rigorous and effective formal education about the media in the UK's 5–14 curricula, which by the early 2000s was showing clear signs of development (Wallis & Buckingham, 2016). However, growing public concern from the 2010s onwards, about the online world of "platforms" and in particular, pre-teens' and teens' use of mobile devices to access them, has given Ofcom's remit a new lease of life. It is widening the scope of its research, broadening its methods, gathering evidence from parents of under-3s, liaising with other sectors and institutions already working in media literacy, and developing new research methods.

In the 21st-century the term "literacy" is being increasingly co-opted in ways that are very different from the 17th-century usage of this word, as "acquainted with letters: educated, learned, polite, liberally educated" – probably what many people nowadays would call "posh" – but certainly related to school-based learning. Now it gets applied to many different fields, and is frequently used merely to emphasise "safety" or "defence."." Its original status was an important set of skills that would enable people to understand and appreciate printed texts and to discriminate amongst them, and although that's how online searches still turn up definitions in those terms, it may not be understood in that way by most of those who now hear it bandied about. As I write this in early 2026, the extensive Wikipedia entry on

"Literacy" is the best quick guide to the numerous current appropriations of the term: it lists 15 different types of "literacy,"," including financial, ecological, social, and health literacies, which thus has the effect of "literacy" being understood in the vaguer sense of "important stuff that you ought to understand."." "Media Literacy" is now primarily associated with debates about social media for under-16s, and with the "screen time rules" promoted by the AAP until 2016. But it seems unlikely that this will ever affect Early Years frameworks and school curricula.

My focus in this book has been on how at least 75% of babies and toddlers – those aged 0–3 who view TV and VOD – do achieve a basic but real moving-image "literacy" by themselves, in the true sense that repeat-viewing and intense concentration enable them to understand and either enjoy or reject what they watch, and to develop the preferences and choices that guide their viewing as they get older. Understanding, judgement, and broad experience must all be developed as part of anyone's ability to enjoy and value an important and complex cultural form. In this book, I have argued for the recognition of 0–3s' achievements in laying the foundations for what could be their later development of moving image media literacy. In a different configuration of departmental responsibilities, the recognition of these achievements could be the basis of a future policy decision to pay more attention to the development of a critical understanding of these media in primary and secondary schooling – perhaps also to some extent in Early Years provision. In my opinion, such a decision would be a great deal more effective than trying to ban children's and under-16's use of "screens."."

England does now have an agency with responsibility for developing the media literacy competencies of England's 3.75 million children under the age of 4: Ofcom. But Ofcom is faced with an enormous task. The prejudices and fears that arise when "children" and "media" are linked in any context make the task of defining and promoting "media literacy" much harder than developing or updating traditional subjects such as maths or history – though I acknowledge that most innovations in the field of education always encounter at least some outraged or pessimistic responses, as can be seen in the results of any online search. Ofcom produces regular reports on their research, the latest being "Children and Parents: Media Use and Attitudes" Report, published at the time of writing in May 2026.

Ofcom defines media literacy as "the ability to use, understand and create media and communications across multiple formats and services." But Ofcom cannot prescribe how such learning could be fostered, or how the resulting competences could be assessed. The breadth and vagueness of their definition is, they say, "deliberately broad, so that it remains relevant in the context of ongoing rapid technological change." This is reasonable, given that a regulatory body can hardly be expected to take on the detailed and complicated task of devising curricula and assessment. But there are no signs that the Department for Education is likely to take this on either. Ofcom does continue to do important research and has now finally taken responsibility for surveying the "media lives" of children aged between 6 months and two years. Their first report on this, in May 2026, was based on "5008 interviews with parents of children aged 6 months to 17-years-old and 3,426 with children themselves aged 8 to 17)" The research is part of their longer-term "Children's Media Lives" study: "a qualitative longitudinal, ethnographic project which has been running since 2014 and complements our quantitative survey data. As far as possible, the research has followed the same children, aged 8–17, interviewing them on camera each year about their media habits and attitudes" (Ofcom, 2026).

I have suggested that we may be beginning to see a greater stylistic diversity in broadcast and online provision for babies and toddlers, thus rewarding 0–3s' curiosity about these media and developing their interest in taking it further. It is possible that by the time you read this, there may be some provision – or at least planning – for good education about moving image media in your country or region, and perhaps even for the 0–3 age-group. By "good," I mean education that recognises and builds on 0–3s' very early learning and enthusiasm, and provides opportunities for children in Early Years settings to discover a wide range of diverse and high-quality moving image media material that might not be widely available through broadcast or online services, but could extend their awareness of these media's capabilities, helping them to enjoy, analyse, and discriminate amongst many styles and genres. I do not mean education that teaches only resistance to false, misleading information or degrading content (important though that obviously is, at least for older children), but education whose central objective is to develop enthusiasm for media content and styles that are honest and truthful, as well as fascinating and beautiful, and the skills to explore, reflect upon – and maybe argue about – the features that can make a text appealing. Three- and four-year-olds already start to become able to identify features – and later maybe also styles or genres – that they like or dislike. As I described in Chapter 11, this is when they start to make more informed judgments about what they watch: by the time they are six or seven, they relish opportunities to talk about these and to share in family-viewing sessions. Understanding and appreciating the good qualities of a cultural form is valuable in itself, as well as being a more effective way of encouraging the rejection of its bad qualities.

In the likely event that no such education is provided or even planned for in the settings where you work, or where your child/ren attend, then you still might want to take on the task of looking for material, whether online or broadcast, that you think would intrigue, or even challenge, the child/ren you are responsible for, whether as a carer or teacher, or as a parent or grandparent in a home context. In the case of older children – three- or four-year-olds for example, they may have already and found, or heard about, a series or a film that they'd like to see. These choices can all lead easily into talking about what they do and don't like about what they have seen, and very often into re-viewing material that they want to understand better. Both initial reactions and re-viewing can lead into conversations about characters they do or don't like, about motivations, characters' appearance, speculation about what might happen in a future episode. Social media threads can also be a good way for Early Years practitioners, parents, and grandparents to find out about programmes and series that they might want to investigate as suitable for babies or toddlers.

When I did the research for this chapter, provision for viewing and talking about moving image media in the Early Years sector was extremely rare, at least in the Anglophone jurisdictions whose policies I have looked at. Although debate does continue in many countries about "media literacy" and how to develop it, for the most part this rarely impinges on formal education, and not at all on Early Years provision. As of the mid 2020s, policy-makers are considering one-off, high-profile, vote-winning actions like banning social media for under-16s, even though that will obviously be almost impossible to administer and manage. But trying to change educational practice or curricula sounds like long-term wishful thinking, as far as the general public is concerned.

The following summary indicates the extent to which references to moving image media are or are not included in Early Years curricula, mainly of Anglophone jurisdictions. Excellent in many ways though they all are, as of early 2026, there is no mention of these media in the Early Years frameworks and curricula in England, Scotland, or Northern Ireland. The curriculum for Wales: Early Years includes "film and digital media" in its "six areas of learning" but admits that in practice, learning about these is currently more likely in schools than in nursery settings.

In the Republic of Ireland, an updated Aistear: The Early Childhood Curriculum Framework was published in 2024. It acknowledges, as most frameworks do, that "babies, toddlers and young children are learning and developing at a pace that exceeds that of any other stage in their lives." It emphasises the centrality of family, languages, meitheal (community spirit of coming together), and cultures in babies, toddlers, and young children's lives. It is the only curriculum framework I have seen that states the child's needs and rights in the first person, as in "I thrive when you recognise and build on my identity, abilities, interests and experiences. You know the different ways I learn and develop and provide relevant, culturally appropriate and meaningful experiences to help me reach my individual potential." It stresses the term "agentic" in defining 0–3s as individuals who "have voice and influence over their own learning." But, although it stresses individual choices and learning, and recognises "art, drama, dance, and music" as an important part of learning, it only mentions "using digital technologies, where developmentally appropriate" and then only as tools to learn about and connect with nature. There is no mention of film, TV, or video, although smartphones are sometimes used by very young children to film plants and/or animals, birds and insects – and each other! Filming can fruitfully interact with a child's viewing experiences to stimulate their imagination and sense of expressive possibilities.

The Program Standards listed by the United States' National Association for the Education of Young Children (NAEYC) are written in slightly more general terms than the British frameworks (given that the more detailed curricula are established within each US state, not at national level) and they make no mention of moving image media. Likewise, the Headstart Program in the USA (https://headstart.gov/curriculum), which provides a useful list of progression stage outcomes in a wide range of developmental areas, does not mention TV or even "screens." To review the Early Years standards and frameworks of every state would have required a much bigger book. I selected four: Minnesota, Colorado, Vermont, and New York, and found that they all have excellent aspirations for diversity, play, creativity, and hands-on activity, and for cultural experiences such as music and drama – but not for film, TV, or video.

New Zealand's He whāriki mātauranga mō ngā mokopuna o Aotearoa/ Early Childhood Curriculum, and Australia's Early Years Learning Framework, are both far more extensive in their discussions of 0–3's needs and learning modes, including much material relating to the specific interests and needs of indigenous communities, but they do not mention moving image media. However, in the Australian Framework's child-centred "Belonging, Being & Becoming" section, the last of 16 bullet points under the heading "Play-based learning and intentionality" does suggest that educators might "facilitate the integration of popular culture, media and digital technologies which add to children's multimodal play." However, the parenting website www.raisingchildren.net.au offers a pageful of largely negative advice about "screen time," "role-modelling healthy habits," and "exposure to screens and digital technology" even though it was updated in December 2024, eight years after the AAP changed its hitherto influential "screen time" rulings.

In South Africa, nearly two-thirds of the country's 4.5 million 0–5-year-olds live in the poorest 40% of households, with 3.5 million in rural areas, some of which have very little infrastructure. The country's "2030 strategy for Early Childhood Development" is therefore primarily concerned with broadening access to Early Years Provision for every child, which in 2026 was still in the early stages of realisation, and did not include any references to moving image media.

The Council of Ministers of Education, Canada (CMEC), published their Early Learning and Development Framework in 2014, a guidance document aiming to present a "pan-Canadian approach to early learning and development ... to support the development of quality early learning programs"

(p. 4) for Canada's ten provinces and three territories. In this document, "early learning" covers birth to eight years old, so is stronger on broad principles than on detail – and contains more pictures than text – concentrating on learning through play as a way of enhancing brain development and leading to "greater social, emotional and academic success." Canada does have numerous small TV channels in different provinces, some of which broadcast their own low-budget programmes for children, although they may well not be shown in primetime.

I also briefly researched two non-Anglophone countries: Denmark, because I had previously collaborated with Danish colleagues in work contexts, and Finland, through later contacts and recommendations. Danish attitudes and policies concerning moving image media for young children are rather different from all the Anglophone countries' curricula. Denmark has a long-established tradition of film production for children, and a development with significance for Early Years was that in 2021 DR, the Danish public service broadcasting corporation, launched a new streaming platform specifically for the 1–3 age range, called Minisjang. The announcement of the platform in 2020 coincided deliberately with the Disney+ launch of their streaming service in Denmark, with which Minisjang is intended to compete (Christensen, 2020). It also coincided with the Danish Ministry of Education launching a "strengthened pedagogical curriculum" for Danish Early Years provision. This covers virtually all Danish children, who between 0 and 6 years attend family day-care (0–2-year-olds), day nursery (0–2-year-olds), or kindergarten (2–5-year-olds) every day. The new curriculum was based on 2018 amendments to the Danish Act on Early Childhood Education and Care and was expected to be implemented by July 2020.

The curriculum document starts with four principles, taken from Section 8(2) of the Act, which are similar in many ways to the principles in several other jurisdictions, but in this case, they lead to a more adventurous follow-up.

Principles

- *View of the child.* Being a child is valuable in itself.
- *Formation and child perspective.* Children aged two and four years, for example, should be heard and be taken seriously as part of the beginning of a formation process and democratic understanding.
- *Play.* Play is valuable in itself and should be a continuous part of an ECEC setting.
- *Learning.* Learning should be understood in a broad sense, and learning takes place, for example, through play, relationships, planned activities, and exploration of nature, *and by being challenged* (my emphasis, because I thought it was unusual and interesting, and relates to my research findings about the determination that some children have, to re-view and make sense of material that they had initially found challenging).

Follow-up

The framework and content of the curriculum includes provision for learning about and with different art forms such as the performing arts, film, painting, music, singing and literature. Aesthetic experiences enable children to share, see themselves in and interpret their own life experience, thoughts and dreams, as well as those of others. At the same time, these experiences have a bodily dimension in which the impressions leave pre-linguistic marks in the form of bodily sensations and experiences. For example, children may feel a tension in their body when they listen to a captivating story, or they may feel joy or sadness when they look at the colours of a painting.

This is the only Early Years curriculum I have seen that mentions film, as well as being the only one that ventures into embodiment theory (Shapiro, 2014). The framework also stipulates that

> the pedagogical learning environment should ensure that all children have many different cultural experiences, as observers as well as active participants, stimulating the children's involvement, imagination, creativity and curiosity, and the learning environment should support the children in gaining experience of using different materials, tools and media.
>
> (Education, 2020)

Finland's 2018–2024 Act on Early Childhood Education and Care (ECEC) is an extensive document that can be found in English at www.finlex.fi/api/media/statute-foreign-language-translation/687728/mainPdf/main.pdf?timestamp=2018-07-12T21%3A00%3A00.000Z. It relates to centre-based, home-based, and "open activities organised in a suitable place," that may be organised by municipalities, private service providers, or in home-based care.

An early childhood education and care plan is drawn up for every child in family day-care and early education centres. It is prepared in cooperation with the personnel, the guardian, and the child. Finnish parents can choose the childcare options for their child when it is between 9 and 10 months old. The Finnish ECEC includes, among many other competences, multi-literacy, cultural and digital competences, interaction, and expression. *Multi-literacy* is a core competence from the viewpoint of interaction and understanding culturally diverse messages and the surrounding world. *Digital competence* is increasingly a part of children's life. It is needed in interaction between people, in operating in society and different digital environments, and in learning. Strengthening digital competence promotes children's educational equality, though I think we could do with more discussion about what "digital competence" actually is, and whether it is or is not the same thing as whatever "digital literacy" is supposed to mean.

In this book, I have preferred to discuss moving image media within a context that is larger than what are usually thought of as "art forms," because for 0–3-year-olds, learning about their own family's culture is always going to be a significant part of their early learning, even when it's not written into Early Years provision. In the majority of families – at least in developed economies – that culture is likely to include, as well as food, clothing, behaviour, jokes, décor – the list is endless! – and of course, watching and enjoying moving image media, at least some of which I would count as "art" in the sense of "works that are appreciated primarily for their beauty or emotional power" (that's my adaptation of the OED definition, and in my opinion, it could include the aesthetic and emotional pleasures of comedy and sport).

Early Years practitioners in Anglophone jurisdictions will not find much in their national or state policies to support the deliberate inclusion of moving image media in their work with 0–3-year-olds. While there is still widespread suspicion and alarm about the alleged effects of TV-watching, the implicit sub-text of most Early Learning frameworks is that the settings may supplement, or perhaps offer alternative activities, for parents who are stressed or struggling. This may be laudable in many ways, but to ignore moving image media completely is to miss another opportunity to build bridges between Early Learning settings and children's home lives. Parents who are sick of multiple re-runs of *Bluey* or *Paw Patrol* are unlikely to complain about their children excitedly talking about a film or series episode that they had seen in nursery and that was different from anything they had ever encountered before. For example, Chris Whitney describes a nursery class that first saw Duriez' 2002 film *Baboon on the Moon* (available in 2026 on Vimeo) in a screening to which parents, carers and siblings had also been invited. The enthusiastic audience response (despite – or perhaps because of – the film's sad ending) initiated numerous follow-up screenings and a proposal from the children to invite the lonely baboon to come and live with them in the classroom. That generated an extended study of the film: copying the baboon's bedroom and kitchen, much activity in creating objects that he would like to have around him when he arrived, and involving several of the parents in these activities (Whitney, 2010).

Of course, families with babies and toddlers in the UK and around the world have for many years been accessing what is probably the most famous public service provider of TV for children: the BBC's CBeebies channel (https://beebs.io/tv-guide/cbeebies/). It is directed mainly at "preschoolers" which usually means ages 3–5, although its breakthrough series for 0–3s, *Teletubbies* and *In the Night Garden* (both from Ragdoll Productions), are also still (in 2026) available. Some producers of TV and VOD production for children now worry about the impact of streaming services offering a vast range advertising-funded material, particularly YouTube Kids. But the BBC is nevertheless now "meeting the audience where it is and putting more of its content on YouTube" ("Bagehot," 2016). Given its generous production budgets, some of which get allocated to co-productions with other public-service broadcasters (as in the case of *Bluey*, for example – see Chapter 10), this means that, "Bagehot" says, "in the process, quality children's programming almost becomes a public good: something freely available, but difficult for the market to provide."

But other sources of public funding, available to a diverse range of producers, is still desirable. At a conference organised by the UK's Children's Media Foundation (CMF) in early 2026, there was much discussion amongst the media professionals present about the need for the renewal of a UK government initiative called the Young Audiences' Content Fund (YACF), which from 2019 to 2022 had included valuable support for production companies making innovative and attractive material for children. During its three-year pilot, the fund had supported the development of 160 TV and film production projects, and commissions that ended up producing 287 hours of new programmes and films, including some that were suitable for 0–3s (Barratt, 2025). The result of YACF's closure means, according to one speaker, that UK TV production for children is now 71% less than it was when the fund was active. Given that the UK Government's 2025 industrial strategy emphasised the potential of the creative sector to act as a "dynamic growth engine" for the larger economy, I'm hoping that by the time you read this, the YACF may have been renewed, although that would require industrial strategists to recognise that young children's cultural experiences do actually matter, even in the long term.

TAKEAWAYS

Further reading

Souza, M. D., & Cabello, P., eds. (2010). *The emerging media toddlers*. Gothenburg: Nordicom: The International Clearinghouse on Children, Youth and Media. A little out of date now, but interesting accounts from Chile, France, the South Pacific, and Sweden, of pre-schoolers' relationships with screen media.

Ofcom publishes a Media Literacy Strategy every three years, at www.ofcom.org.uk/media-use-and-attitudes/media-literacy/ofcoms-three-year-media-literacy-strategy.

The Children's Media Foundation (www.thechildrensmediafoundation.org/) publishes an annual Yearbook on the state of children's media provision and the key issues and news about children's media. It campaigns to improve the funding and regulation of children's content, and to prevent harmful material and influences from reaching children and young people.

References

"Bagehot." (2016, March 21, 2026). CBeebies or Barbarism! *The Economist.*

Barratt, J. (2025). *Young audiences content fund pilot: End-of-term evaluation: Supplementary update.* Retrieved from London: www.bfi.org.uk/; https://core-cms.bfi.org.uk/media/41790/download

Christensen, C. L. (2020). Danish children's content for 1-3-year olds and the importance of national platforms like the Danish Broadcasting Corporation, DR. Retrieved from https://cstonline.net/danish-childrens-content-for-1-3-year-olds-and-the-importance-of-national-platforms-like-the-danish-broadcasting-corporation-dr/

Education, M. o. (2020). *The strengthened pedagogical curriculum: Framework and content.* Copenhagen: Danish Government.

Ofcom. (2026). *Children and Parents: Media Use and Attitudes Report 2025-6.* Retrieved from London, UK: www.ofcom.org.uk/siteassets/resources/documents/research-and-data/media-literacy-research/children/2026-children-and-parents-report/children-and-parents-media-use-and-attitudes-report-2025-6.pdf?v=418231&utm_medium=email&utm_campaign=Childrens%20media%20literacy%20research%20published%20today&utm_content=Childrens%20media%20literacy%20research%20published%20today+CID_4ab35f73b1338264c84414a1ed85ae4a&utm_source=media%20literacy%20bulletin&utm_term=Children%20and%20Parents%20Media%20Use%20and%20Attitudes

Shapiro, L. A. (Ed.) (2014). *The Routledge handbook of embodied cognition.* Abingdon: Routledge.

Wallis, R., & Buckingham, D. (2013). Arming the citizen-consumer: The invention of 'media literacy' within UK communications policy. *European Journal of Communication, 28*(5). https://doi.org/10.1177/0267323113483605

Wallis, R., & Buckingham, D. (2016). Media literacy: The UK's undead cultural policy. *International Journal of Cultural Policy.* Retrieved from http://dx.doi.org/10.1080/10286632.2016.1229314

Whitney, C. (2010). A learning journey. In C. Bazalgette (Ed.), *Teaching media in primary schools* (pp. 75–84). London: Sage.

Conclusion

My purpose in writing this book has been to propose and describe a new way of thinking about 0–3s experiences with the moving image media of television, video, and film. It's different from most of the other writing on this topic, for two reasons. First, it draws on close observations over an extended period. My "sample" of just two children may be scorned as much too limited, and liable to bias for being a study of my own grandchildren. I think that would be a reasonable objection if I were gathering evidence to support a theory or to answer a question, but that wasn't my purpose.

I started with the vague idea of "looking at what happens," but it turned out to be a process of generating a proposition, starting from what I already knew from my long experience in media education: that moving image media have their own "language" through which they tell stories, provide information, and circulate ideas. This must mean that children have to learn, from a very early age if they have the opportunities, how to understand the stories that moving image media tell. And they must do this largely on their own: parents and older siblings may drop hints, but babies and toddlers have to learn that language by themselves. My research showed me the observable aspects of that learning. I didn't see the beginning of it, because, like the majority of British babies (Marsh et al., 2005), the twins had been viewing TV since they were three months old (though of course I had viewed with them many times during that first year). But I have talked with many parents and grandparents about those early stages and visited social media threads that discussed babies, toddlers, TV, and YouTube. The fact that babies and toddlers are fascinated by moving images from the first time they see them, together with the fact that, as time goes by, they keep moving on to more complex material, are the evidence that learning must be happening.

Secondly, I was shocked by the poor quality of the voluminous research that has underpinned the mantra "no TV before 2 years old" and the "screen time" notion. More recently, I've been cheered by critiques of that research (Duch et al., 2013; Etchells, 2024), and the American Association of Pediatrics modification of its "screen time" rules (AAP, 2016). And I have watched with interest the justifiable shift of public attention towards teenagers, mobile

DOI: 10.4324/9781003751236-14

devices, social media propaganda, and the critiques of knee-jerk responses such as bans.

This book is primarily for Early Years practitioners and carers, but I hope it will also interest many parents and grandparents. My aim is to provoke new thinking and greater confidence in children's immense capacity for learning. And I hope that you share my belief in the value of moving image media in our culture, as one of our major sources of information, ideas and, of course, pleasure.

References

AAP. (2016). American Academy of Pediatrics Announces New Recommendations for Children's Media Use [Press release].

Duch, H., Fisher, E. M., Ensari, I., & Harrington, A. (2013). Screen time use in children under 3 years old: A systematic review of correlates. *The International Journal of Behavioral Nutrition and Physical Activity, 10*(1).

Etchells, P. (2024). *Unlocked: The real science of screen time (and how to spend it better)*. London: Platkus.

Marsh, J., Brooks, G., Hughes, J., Ritchie, L., Roberts, S., & Wright, K. (2005). *Digital beginnings: Young children's use of popular culture, media and new technologies*. Retrieved from Sheffield: www.researchgate.net/publication/265183910_Digital_beginnings_Young_children%27s_use_of_popular_culture_media_and_new_technologies (accessed 08-11-2021).

Index

For Product Safety Concerns and Information please contact our EU representative GPSR@taylorandfrancis.com Taylor & Francis Verlag GmbH, Kaufingerstraße 24, 80331 München, Germany

Batch number: 10726548

Printed by Printforce, the Netherlands